# color
# me
# younger

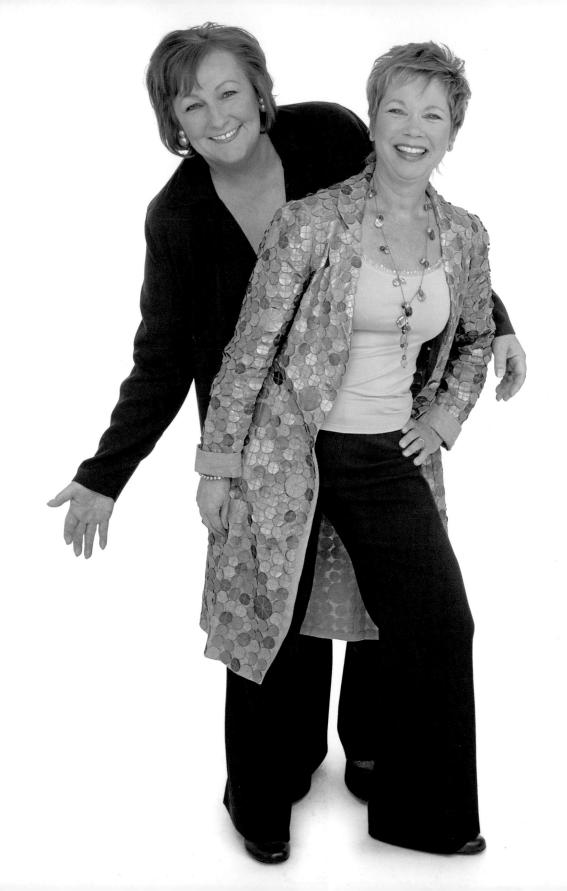

# color
# me
# younger

with colour**me**beautiful

Veronique Henderson
Pat Henshaw

hamlyn

*This book is dedicated to all those women who have shown charm and a zest for life in the face of adversity. Thank you for your inspiration.*

An Hachette UK Company
www.hachette.co.uk

First published in Great Britain in 2008 by
Hamlyn, a division of Octopus Publishing Group Ltd
2–4 Heron Quays, London E14 4JP
www.octopusbooksusa.com

This edition published in 2009

Distributed in the U.S. and Canada by
Octopus Books USA:
c/o Hachette Book Group
237 Park Avenue
New York NY 10017

Every effort has been made to reproduce the
colors in this book accurately; however, the
printing process can lead to some discrepancies. The
color samples provided should be used as a guideline
only.

ISBN: 978-0-600-61961-1

A CIP catalog record for this book is available
from the Library of Congress.

Printed and bound in China

10 9 8 7 6 5 4 3 2 1

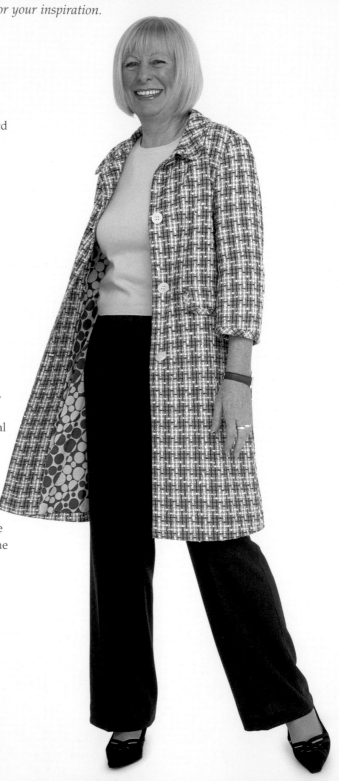

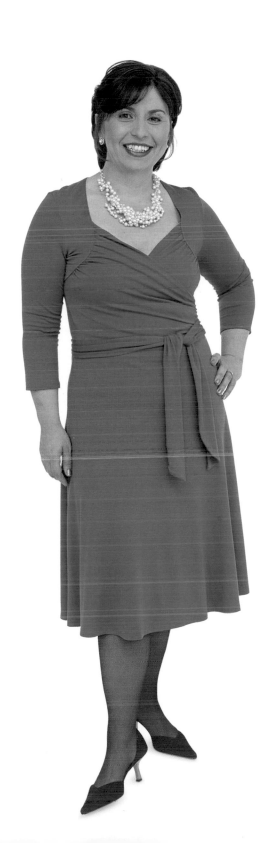

# Contents

# Introduction

In our time, we—women now in our 40s, 50s, 60s, and beyond—have been hippies; we invented the miniskirt, and we have been punks, too. We were teenagers in the 1950s, '60s, and '70s; we listened to rock and pop and now we know that life begins at 40, at 50, at 60, and beyond.

Every phase we go through calls for some rethinking. We reassess who we are and how others perceive us. We change our outlook on life as we grow older and so, inevitably, do we change our inner makeup and our outer appearance. Our skin ages, our hair grays, our waists thicken, and we seek new ways of dressing to look our best. But should this mean that we must automatically abandon all ideas of youth and vitality? No! We are still attractive, we are still sexy, and we still need to feel good about ourselves.

## The older you

There is nothing wrong with your laughter and expression lines. They show that you have lived and enjoy life to the full. The telltale signs of aging are nothing to be ashamed of. Rather, you must embrace them and accept them as the new you—a confident, beautiful, mature woman. Cosmetic surgery, with its promise of eternal youth, may seem to be an attractive option, but treatment tends to be expensive, invasive, and can end in disappointment. Why take the risk, when you can maintain a youthful appearance just by taking care of yourself and choosing the right clothes to wear?

## The younger you

Based on the practices at **colour me beautiful**, this book shows women in their 40s, 50s, 60s, and beyond how to stay looking younger while acknowledging the fact that they are growing older. Depending on the natural coloring of your hair, skin, and eyes, the book advises you what colors to wear, how to apply makeup, how to style and color your hair, and how to dress to suit your figure, lifestyle, and personality. Each chapter works toward giving you the confidence to create a complete look that makes you appear and feel youthful and radiant, whatever your age.

"There is never anything new in fashion. It just repeats itself in different ways."
Vivienne Westwood

## About **colour me beautiful**

Established over 25 years ago, **colour me beautiful** is recognized as the world's leading image consultancy, with over 1,000 studios worldwide. Since its inception, **colour me beautiful** consultants have color- and style-analyzed millions of women (and men), offering up-to-date advice on achieving a confident self-image. The overwhelming response to their work—evident in the feedback of the thousands of satisfied clients—is that once a woman finds the colors, makeup, hairstyle, and style of clothing that work for her, she looks and feels younger, has more confidence, and just wants to keep on having fun and enjoying life.

If this is something that appeals to you (and why wouldn't it?), read on to discover how you can look better than ever simply by dressing to show off your shape and giving your hair and makeup a new lease on life. See how easy it is to remain feminine and attractive in your 40s, 50s, 60s, and beyond—confident in who and what you are, positive in outlook, and youthful in spirit.

**"A woman doesn't learn to dress well until she is over 35."**
Christian Dior

# Younger colors

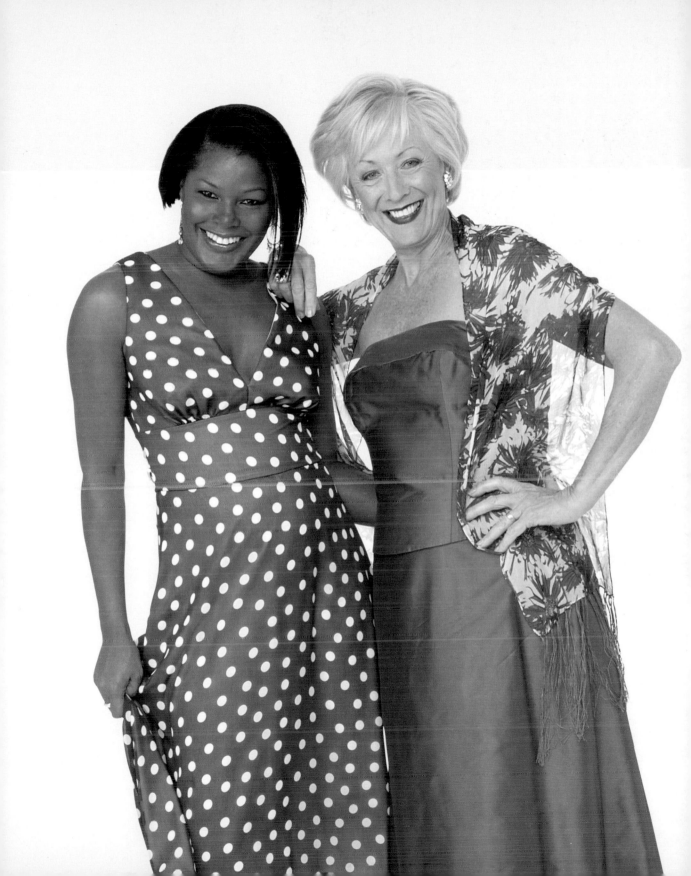

# All about color

From the time you wake up in the morning to the time you go back to bed at night, and even in your dreams, you are surrounded by color—it is everywhere and in everything you do.

Whether you know it or not, color influences the way you feel and how you look. Light colors energize you while dark colors slow you down. Your mood is uplifted by clear yellow and orange, while darker, richer colors, such as brown and forest green, are warm and comforting. And so it goes.

When it comes to the clothes you wear, you may well have a very good idea of the colors that are most flattering for you or that seem to suit you best, but do you know which colors to avoid? Just as you might find a colorful scene uplifting and pleasing to the eye—say a prize-winning garden in full bloom—you, and the colors you wear, will have a similar effect on the people you meet. And if you understand which colors complement your coloring you will receive many more compliments because you are pleasing to the eye. You'll please yourself, too, when looking in a mirror, and you will feel more positive in the process.

**Next time someone asks you if you are feeling ill or are "off color," think about whether it might just be a case of wearing the wrong color near your face.**

## You and color

Your coloring—your hair, skin, and eyes—take on a different appearance, depending on what you are wearing and, specifically, on the colors you choose to wear near your face. If you select a color that harmonizes with your own coloring, it will reflect similar tones and shades in your face, enhancing your natural look. Choose an inappropriate color, however, and you run the risk of casting dark shadows across your face, emphasizing the lines that age you, and making your skin, hair, and eyes look dull.

By subtly changing the tone of a color, wearing it with or less contrast, or even wearing it away from the face, you can make yourself look younger and healthier. Even just changing your favorite lipstick color can make an enormous difference. And knowing the right tints to add to your hair can ensure that you continue to keep your youthful glow.

## Color theory

The **colour me beautiful** methodology is based on the Munsell system, which describes color as having the following three characteristics:
• Depth: from light to dark, where 0 is black and 10 is white, with all the grays in between. Every color can be described in these terms.
• Undertone: from warm (yellow-toned) to cool (blue-toned). Each color in the spectrum can be said to have a warm or cool undertone. For example, a cool (blue) red has a more plummy color to it, while a warm (yellow) red is more orange.
• Clarity: from clear to soft, depending on how

much gray there is in a color. The less gray, the brighter (clearer) the color, while more gray makes a color muted, or soft.

At **colour me beautiful** these elements are used to define the six main dominant characteristics when describing people: light, deep, warm, cool, clear, and soft, depending primarily on the color of their eyes, hair, and skin. Of course, there are many variations to these basic types, but it is important to understand which of them describes you best. Then you can make informed choices when it comes to wearing color successfully.

It is also worth bearing in mind that the primary elements of your own coloring—particularly your hair—change with the aging process, sometimes dramatically. So, although you may have had your colors done in the past, it is important that you look at yourself again in your 40s, 50s, 60s, and beyond to make sure you are wearing the right shades for a younger-looking you. For some of you this aging process might mean adding a semi-permanent tint to your hair to keep your dominant, while others may decide to help nature along and completely change your dominant characteristic.

Barbra Streisand in her 30s, with dark hair and bright eyes, was a perfect clear.

Today Barbra Streisand's hair is lighter, her eyes softer, and she has matured beautifully into a soft.

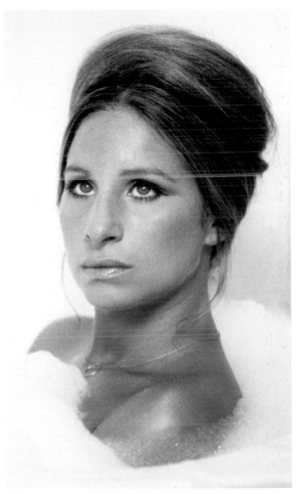

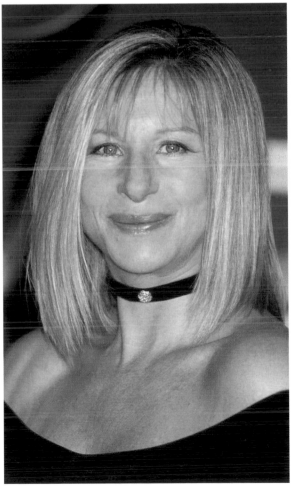

# Finding your right colors

Your first step to looking younger is to identify your dominant color characteristics. This will make you better able to choose the right colors to wear whether you are in your 40s, 50s, 60s, or beyond.

## What is your dominant?

Opposite are the main physical characteristics for each of the six color types described on page 11. Be honest with yourself, and consider the type that best describes you as you are right now, and not how you were five, ten, or twenty years ago. It is not always easy to be objective about your own coloring and you may be surprised to find that your dominant coloring characteristic has changed. Once you know your dominant, turn to the pages given to find the best color palette for a younger look, whatever age you are. If you find that you are a combination of two dominants, look at the soft dominant again.

### A note about black

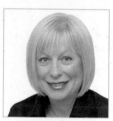
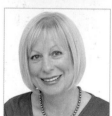
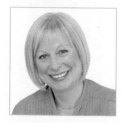

For most women, black is a wardrobe staple. Not only can you wear it with most colors, but it is also perceived as being slimming, and for some women this is true, as long as it is worn in the right place.

As you grow older, however, you should think about whether black is still a flattering color to wear near the face if you want to achieve a younger look. To find out for yourself, simply hold a black garment near your face to see if there are any shadows under your chin. Only some of the coloring types, or dominants, discussed on the following pages can still wear black successfully. For those of you who don't have black in your color palettes, consider using it below the waist, with a low neckline, or with accessories (necklaces, scarves) in your right colors.

If you can't bring yourself to give up on your black jacket or coat, remember to wear one of your most flattering colors near your face so that the light of that color reflects on your face, making you look younger. An alternative to solid black is to use it in a fabric that softens the color, such as tweed, velvet, suede, or burnout fabrics. For example, using a black-and-white tweed mix will give you a softer gray color. Sheer fabrics and lace are other excellent examples of how to wear black successfully near your face.

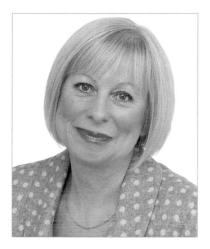

### The light dominant
- You have light blonde or white hair.
- You have light blue or green eyes.
- Your skin is porcelain and delicate.
- Go to pages 14–21.

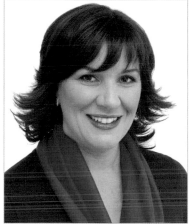

### The deep dominant
- You have black to dark brown hair.
- You have dark brown eyes.
- Your skin is anything from very dark to very pale.
- Go to pages 22–29.

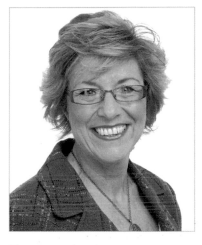

### The warm dominant
- You have strawberry blonde to auburn hair.
- Your eyes are blue, green, or hazel.
- Your skin is freckled or golden.
- Go to pages 30–37.

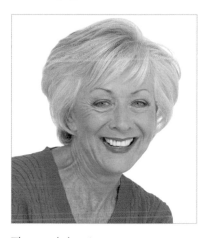

### The cool dominant
- You have ash blonde, black, or gray hair.
- Your eyes are blue, gray, or cool brown.
- You have cool (blue or pink) undertones to the skin.
- Go to pages 38–45.

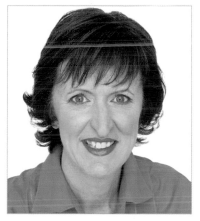

### The clear dominant
- You have medium to dark brown hair.
- Your eyes are bright blue, green, or topaz.
- You have a clear, fresh complexion.
- Go to pages 46–53.

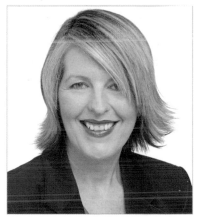

### The soft dominant
- You have mousy, often highlighted, hair.
- Your eyes are soft brown, green or blue (or a combination of all three).
- You have a neutral complexion.
- Go to pages 54–61.

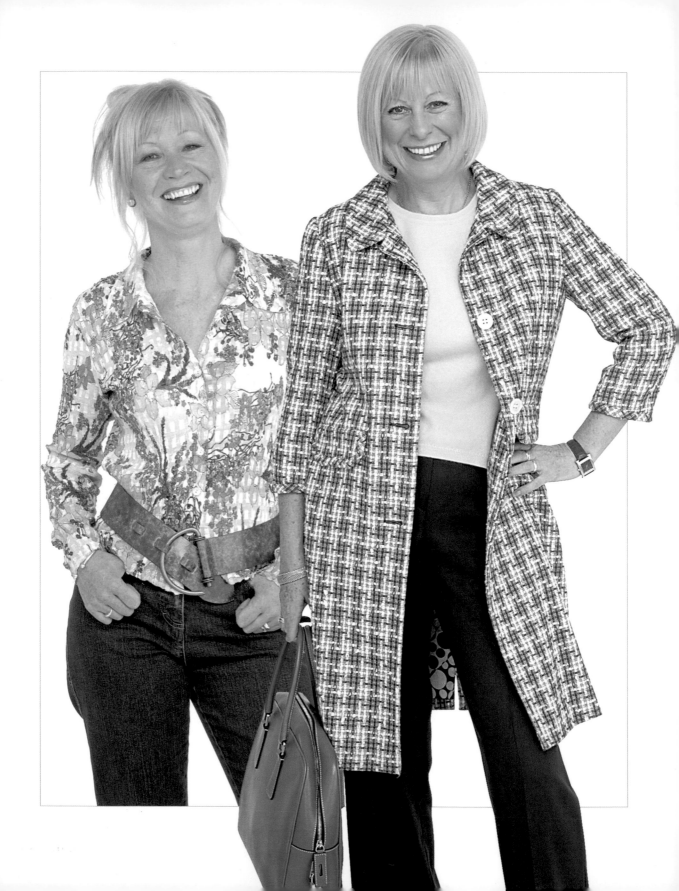

# Light

If most or all of your color characteristics fall into this category, your overall appearance is likely to be pale and delicate, with naturally light hair, eyes, and skin tones.

You have blonde, silver-gray, or even white hair. The texture of your hair may be fine and prone to thinning with age. Your eyebrows are pale and, in some instances, virtually nonexistent. Your eyelashes also tend to be very pale and sometimes quite sparse. Your skin is porcelain in color and could be sensitive—some broken capillaries may start to appear now. Your eyes are pale and may even be lighter in color than they were several years ago.

hair tends to fade as you age, and if your skin has developed some rosy tones, wear colors with a cool (or blue-based) undertone, such as peacock, for a younger look.

### Clarity: clear or soft
If your eyes are bright and clear, use the brighter, more vibrant, colors of your palette such as blush pink and light teal. If your eyes have softened try dusty rose or sky blue.

## Key elements of your colors
There are a number of colors that you can wear well, referred to as your "palette" (see pages 16–17). When you assemble an outfit, however, always consider the following key elements.

### Depth: from light to medium
Your navies and grays should be as light as possible; you are better off using pewters and taupes to replace black, if appropriate.

### Undertone: warm or cool
If your hair is golden blonde and you have a few freckles, use colors that have a warm (or yellow) undertone, like apple green. If the warmth in your

## Accessories for a younger look
Don't underestimate the role that accessories can play in your look. Hats, scarves, footwear, bags, and jewelry can all be used to give an outfit that extra style, while bringing your wardrobe staples right up to date. Use them to break up simple lines, to accentuate your best features, and to add bold color or style without overpowering your look.

Complete an outfit with lighter-colored shoes and bags. (A black bag and shoes with a light taupe outfit will overwhelm the look). Similarly, keep the colors of your jewelry light (for example, citrine, aquamarine, amethyst). Pearls, either earrings or necklaces, are always a great standby to lift medium to dark colors.

As a light dominant, always keep light colors near your face.

# The light palette

The colors listed here offer a good, basic range of what you should be looking for in order to stay looking young and radiant. Women in their 50s or 60s and beyond may find that their colors are lighter and cooler than in their 40s (see pages 19–21).

## Neutrals

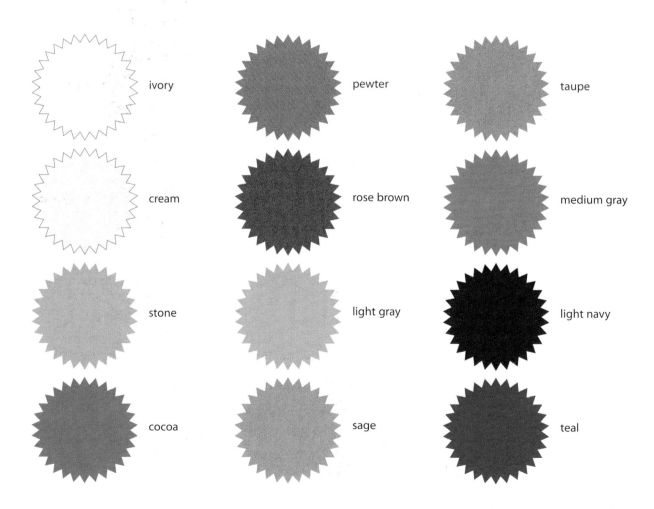

ivory

pewter

taupe

cream

rose brown

medium gray

stone

light gray

light navy

cocoa

sage

teal

## Lights

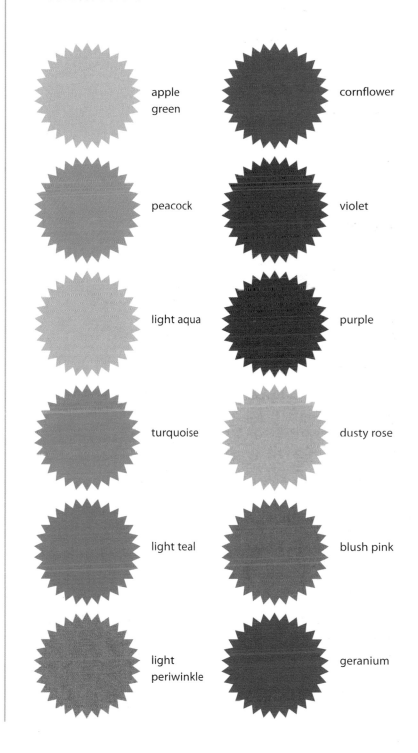

soft white

pastel pink

light apricot

primrose

mint

sky blue

## Fashion colors

apple green

peacock

light aqua

turquoise

light teal

light periwinkle

cornflower

violet

purple

dusty rose

blush pink

geranium

# Looking younger with the light palette

## Using your palette for a younger you

The light palette is a fresh and feminine one, with colors that are very flattering for the mature woman. Careful use of the neutral colors is important for those of you who have a formal business wardrobe. Successful use of colors such as medium gray, taupe, and lighter shades of navy, will always give you a more youthful look.

## The good news

Of all the dominants, you can have the most fun shopping in the spring and summer months, when light and pastel shades are abundant. You can also choose from a wide range of fabrics when selecting what to wear. Keep in mind that it makes sense to choose machine-washable pieces, however, because lighter shades have a tendency to get grubby quicker. The best news for you is that the light and clean colors of this palette will reflect onto your face, minimizing any dark shadows around the eyes and mouth.

## The bad news

Avoid wearing two dark colors together—this will just overpower your natural coloring. Your biggest challenge will be buying a winter coat, since the majority of them come in dark colors; camel is a great option—just make sure it doesn't match your hair too closely!

## The rules

✓ Always wear a light color near the face.

✓ You may wear two light colors together.

✓ When wearing medium to dark shades from your palette, always add a light contrasting color; this can be in the form of jewelry, shoes, or scarves.

✓ Your skin is fine and delicate, so wear as light a foundation as possible.

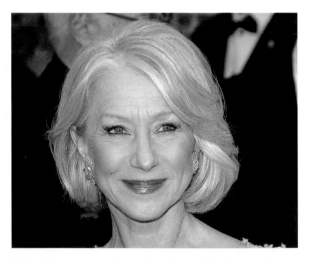

Joely Richardson is a natural golden blonde and a great example of a light in her 40s.

Helen Mirren may not always have been a light but now her warm gray hair and pale eyebrows make her a classic example.

# Looking younger
## in your 40s

Women in their 40s may find that their coloring has started to fade a little, and that this is probably more noticeable in their hair than in their complexion. Here's what works for you.

## Light colors you should use next to your face

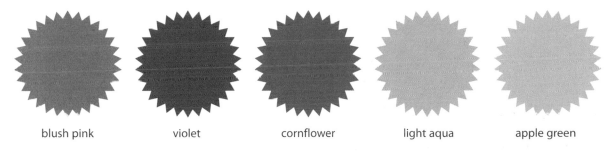

| blush pink | violet | cornflower | light aqua | apple green |

## Light color combinations to try

| rose brown | light navy | petrol | pewter | light denim |

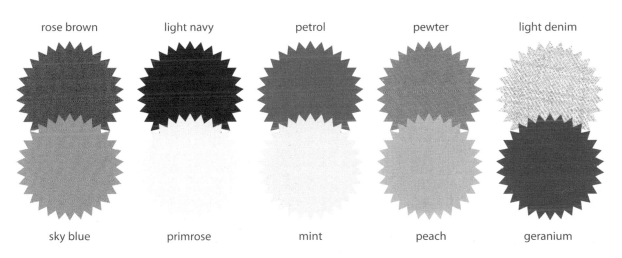

| sky blue | primrose | mint | peach | geranium |

# Looking younger
# in your 50s

If you are in your 50s, you may have noticed that your natural coloring is cooler now, and has more pink tones appearing on your skin (possibly caused by broken capillaries). You may consider a tint in your hair.

## Light colors you should use next to your face

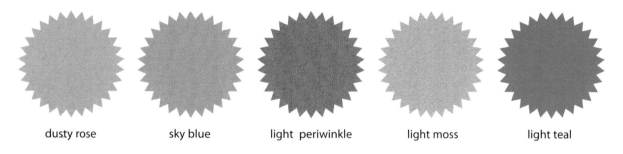

| dusty rose | sky blue | light periwinkle | light moss | light teal |

## Light color combinations to try

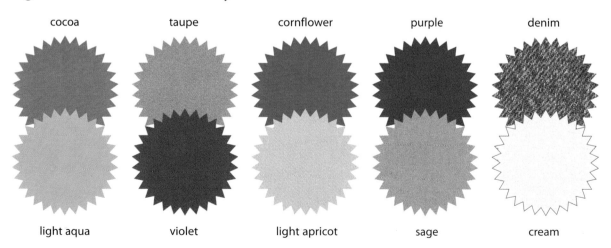

| cocoa | taupe | cornflower | purple | denim |
| light aqua | violet | light apricot | sage | cream |

# Looking younger
## in your 60s and beyond

Your coloring may be fairly delicate now, so avoid strong contrasting color combinations. Look for colors that are a bit lighter and cooler than those in the basic palette on pages 16–17.

## Light colors you should use next to your face

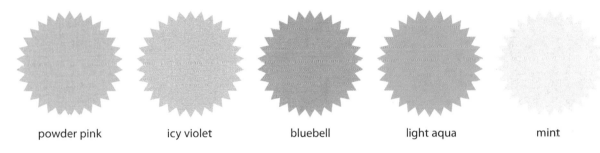

powder pink     icy violet     bluebell     light aqua     mint

## Light color combinations to try

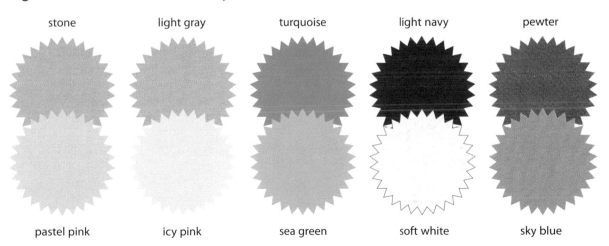

stone     light gray     turquoise     light navy     pewter

pastel pink     icy pink     sea green     soft white     sky blue

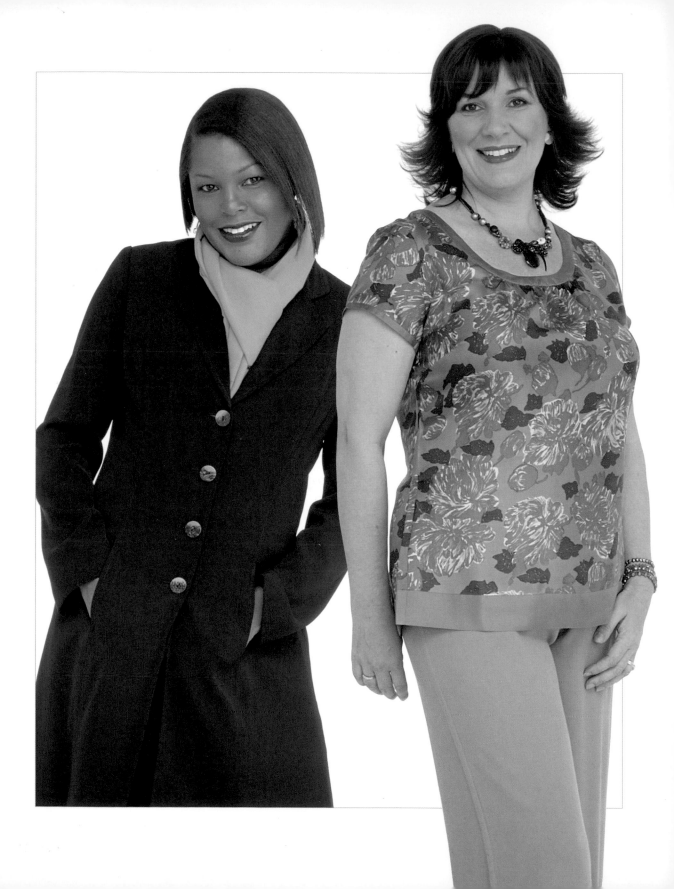

# Deep

If most or all of your color characteristics fall into this category, your overall appearance is likely to be rich and strong.

Your look has always been dominated by your dark eyes and hair, and the secret to looking younger is to maintain this look for as long as it is appropriate. The biggest challenge is your changing hair color, which inevitably lightens your look. Of the six types, you are more likely than the others to need to change your dominant if you are in your 50s or 60s and beyond—probably to soft. The alternative is to consider enhancing your natural hair color as you age. A good guide as to whether you need to do this is to see what is happening to your eyebrows. If they are lighter than your hair, it is time for a change.

## Key elements of your colors

There are a number of colors that you can wear well, referred to as your "palette" (see pages 24–25). When you assemble an outfit, however, always consider the following key elements.

### Depth: from light to dark

You can wear light and dark colors together—for example, chocolate and lime—or just dark colors on their own—for example, pine and dark navy.

### Undertone: warm or cool

If you have warm/red tones to your hair, warmer (yellow-based) shades such as bittersweet are best

worn near your face. If you are beginning to get natural highlights, you might consider adding plum shades to your hair, and then the cooler (blue-based) colors are more complementary near your face (try burgundy).

### Clarity: clear or soft

In your 40s and early 50s have the confidence to wear bright, clear shades such as blush pink or cornflower. In your 60s and beyond, you might want to change to rust or amethyst.

## Accessories for a younger look

Don't underestimate the role that accessories can play in your look. Hats, scarves, footwear, bags, and jewelry can all be used to give an outfit that extra style, while bringing your wardrobe staples right up to date. Use them to break up simple lines, to accentuate your best features, and to add color or style without overpowering your look.

Black, navy, and brown shoes or bags will always work for you if you are cautious about using color in your wardrobe. However, this is also your opportunity for injecting some color. Wear beads and jewelry in tigereye, garnet, amber, ruby, and jet with metals and natural materials such as wood and leather.

Play with color combinations. A dark coat with a bright scarf or outfits in medium shades with jewelry in deeper tones will be a winner on you.

# The deep palette

The colors listed here offer a good, basic range of what you should be looking for in order to stay looking young and radiant. Women in their 50s or 60s and beyond may find that their colors are lighter and cooler than in their 40s (see pages 27–29).

## Neutrals

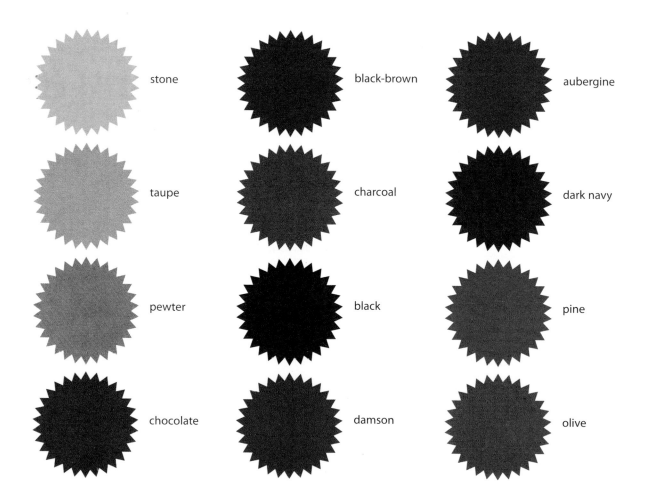

stone

black-brown

aubergine

taupe

charcoal

dark navy

pewter

black

pine

chocolate

damson

olive

## Lighter colors

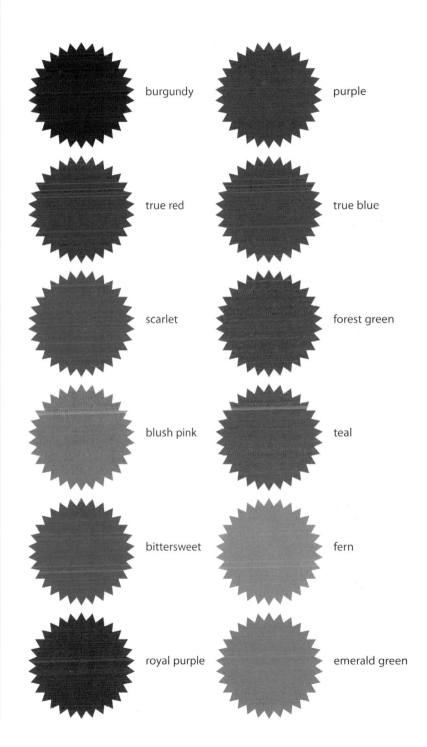

soft white

ivory

primrose

lime

turquoise

cornflower

## Fashion colors

burgundy

purple

true red

true blue

scarlet

forest green

blush pink

teal

bittersweet

fern

royal purple

emerald green

# Looking younger
## with the **deep palette**

### Using your palette for a younger you

You are probably used to wearing strong, deep and rich colors. You might want to consider combining these tones with colors that are lighter or softer near your face, since darker shades may now emphasize expression lines. By adding shades of red and pink you soften the effects of dark colors on the face and achieve a more youthful look.

You may need to change your hair color, since dark hair looks unnatural with age. If you follow this route, you will need to return to page 13 to determine your dominant.

### The good news

You have an abundance of wonderful shades in your palette. Wear them with confidence, and you can continue to look stunning for many years. You are also one of the lucky few who can wear black (although you may need to be cautious here). Wear it with other colors in your palette, choose black accessories, and you will always look coordinated.

### The bad news

Unfortunately, now is the time to give up the black eyeliner; you will find charcoal a much more flattering alternative. Also, if you find that you are adding more makeup or color when you wear black, you should probably think about moving it away from your face.

### The rules

✓ Don't wear two light colors together.

✓ If you like pastel shades, wear them as a contrast with darker colors.

✓ In the summer, wear bright colors near your face and not whites, taupes, or beiges.

✓ When wearing just one dark color on its own, use accessories to lift the color.

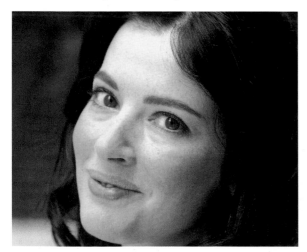

Nigella Lawson is the perfect example of a woman in her 40s who is a deep.

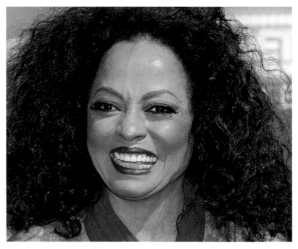

Diana Ross keeps her hair a striking black, while complementing it by wearing strong, rich colors.

# Looking younger in your 40s

Many women in their 40s find that their coloring loses some of its intensity and that they need to adjust the color of their clothes to remain young looking. Here's what to look for.

## Deep colors you should use next to your face

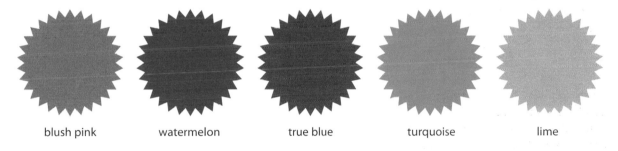

| blush pink | watermelon | true blue | turquoise | lime |

## Deep color combinations to try

| black | aubergine | taupe | true red | black-brown |

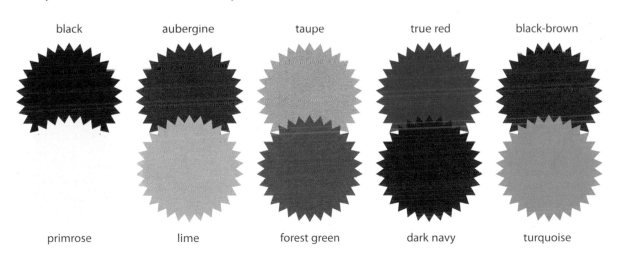

| primrose | lime | forest green | dark navy | turquoise |

# Looking younger
## in your 50s

If you are in your 50s, you can continue to wear your color palette, but think about adding texture to your colors in order to diffuse their intensity and soften the look (see page 55). This may be the time to consider tinting your hair.

## Deep colors you should use next to your face

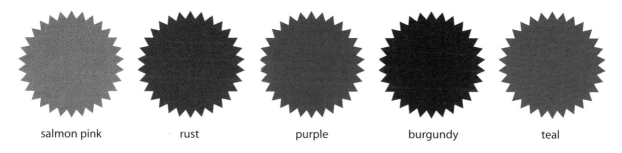

| salmon pink | rust | purple | burgundy | teal |

## Deep color combinations to try

| charcoal | chocolate | damson | forest green | true blue |

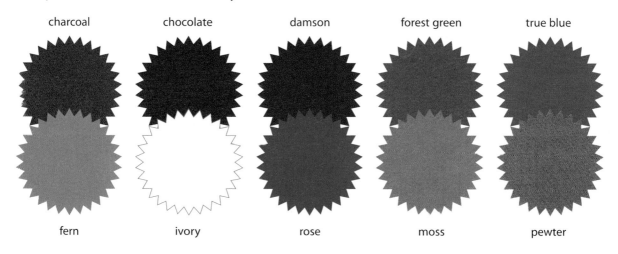

| fern | ivory | rose | moss | pewter |

# Looking younger
# in your 60s and beyond

A number of women in their 60s and beyond will find themselves moving to another dominant in order to accommodate their lighter characteristics. If you remain **deep**, adjust your palette to reflect the cooler tones in your hair and skin.

## Deep colors you should use next to your face

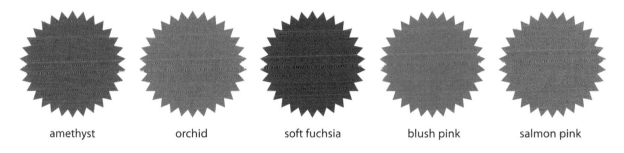

| amethyst | orchid | soft fuchsia | blush pink | salmon pink |

## Deep color combinations to try

| olive | royal purple | dark navy | pine | burgundy |

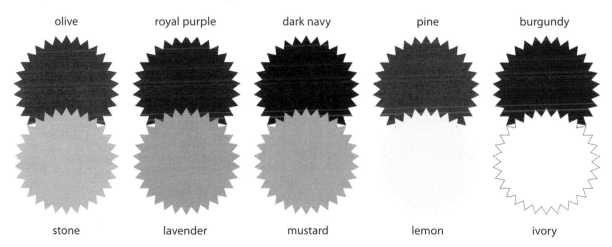

| stone | lavender | mustard | lemon | ivory |

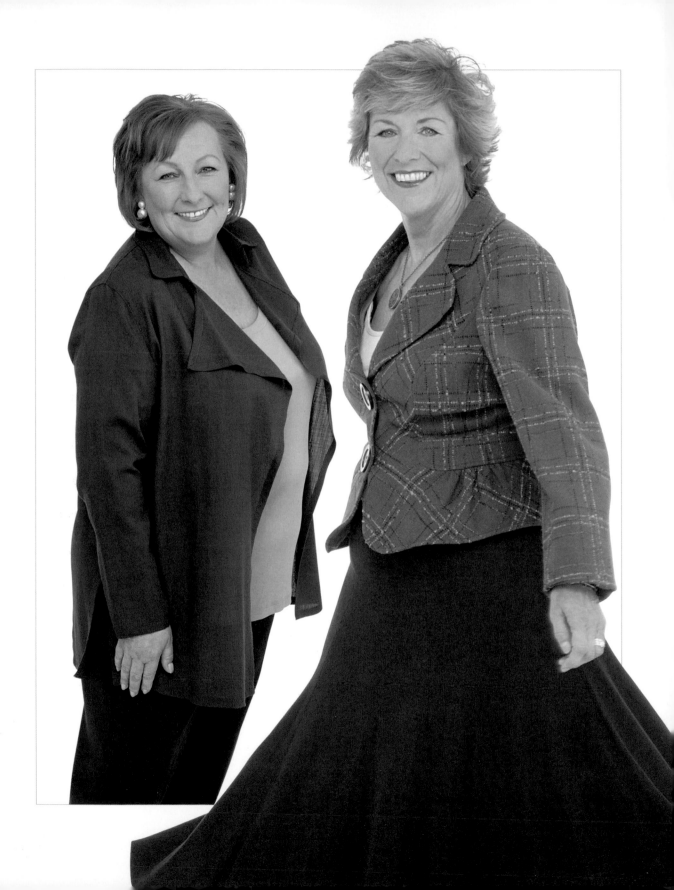

# Warm

If most or all of your color characteristics fall into this category, your overall appearance is likely to be golden, with an aura of warmth.

Whether your eyes are brown, green, or blue, all the colors you wear need to have a warm (yellow-based) undertone. Your hair may vary from deep auburn to light strawberry blonde. If your skin tone is porcelain with freckles, your eyebrows and eyelashes are likely to be pale. If you have deep, golden skin your eyebrows may be dark in color. To keep your youthful look, consider enhancing your hair color now that it shows signs of gray.

## Key elements of your colors

There are a number of colors that you can wear well, referred to as your "palette" (see pages 32–33). When you assemble an outfit, however, always consider the following key elements.

### Depth: from light to medium

You need to balance the depth of your colors with the depth of your hair. The lighter the hair, the lighter the shades you should wear. With darker hair and eyes, you will be able to wear the darker tones of the palette.

### Undertone: warm

All the colors you wear need to have a yellow base. Therefore, when wearing light navy and

charcoal, for example, warm them up with yellows and salmons.

### Clarity: clear or soft

Those of you who have bright green or blue eyes will look stunning in the clearer shades such as coral and lime. If you have brown or topaz eyes, try softer shades, such as mahogany or rust, near your face.

## Accessories for a younger look

Don't underestimate the role that accessories can play in your look. Hats, scarves, footwear, bags, and jewelry can all be used to give an outfit that extra style, while bringing your wardrobe staples right up to date. Use them to break up simple lines, to accentuate your best features, and to add color or style without overpowering your look.

To complement your warm tones, try bronze, tan, and brown shoes and bags. When it comes to jewelry, natural materials are great for you, as well as copper, bronze, and beads. Colors can include jade, topaz, amber, peridot, coral, and aquamarine. Creamy or apricot-toned pearls are perfect, especially when worn with your neutrals.

With so many shades of brown available, brown is now the new black for a warm. Have fun teaming it with all the other shades of your palette.

# The warm palette

The colors listed here offer a good, basic range of what you should be looking for in order to stay looking young and radiant. Women in their 50s or 60s and beyond may find that their colors are lighter and cooler than in their 40s (see pages 35–37).

## Neutrals

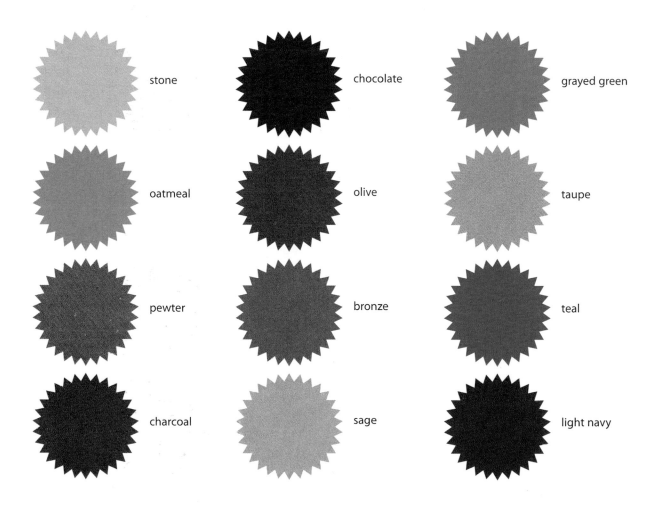

stone

chocolate

grayed green

oatmeal

olive

taupe

pewter

bronze

teal

charcoal

sage

light navy

## Lighter colors

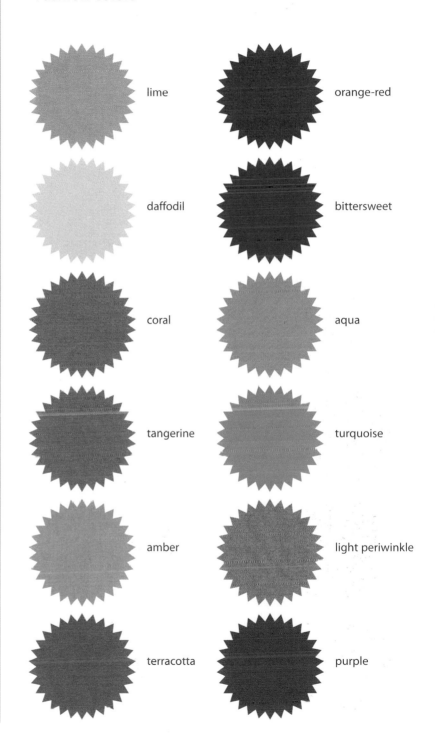

soft white

cream

apricot

light apricot

primrose

mint

## Fashion colors

lime

daffodil

coral

tangerine

amber

terracotta

orange-red

bittersweet

aqua

turquoise

light periwinkle

purple

# Looking younger
## with the **warm palette**

## Using your palette for a younger you

Using yellow-based colors near your face will cast warm tones over the skin, which will flatter and harmonize your complexion. The darker, neutral colors in your palette—charcoal, chocolate, light navy, and olive—need to be complemented with the lighter shades near your face.

### The good news

You are lucky, because your fashion colors add invigorating warmth even on the dullest day. Just by adding a colorful top, scarf, or piece of jewelry, you will bring a fun, youthful look to any outfit you wear. The best news is that your graying hair will take well to tinting, because your base color will retain some of its natural red.

### The bad news

You have to be cautious when selecting any pink clothes. Pink may be a color you find comforting, but yours must remain a yellow-based one like a coral or apricot, rather than a blue-based one, which will be too cool for your looks. You will also need to think about replacing your black with charcoal or chocolate, which are much more flattering when worn near your face.

### The rules

✓ Make the most of your fabulous hair color with good conditioning and a current hairstyle.

✓ Either wear bright, contrasting shades or use color tone-on-tone.

✓ Always wear really warm tones near your face when wearing light navy and charcoal.

✓ Banish any blue-based pinks from your closet and makeup bag.

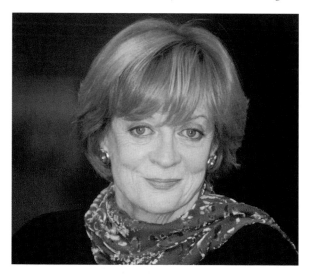

Maggie Smith in her 60s has kept her hair color rich and warm looking.

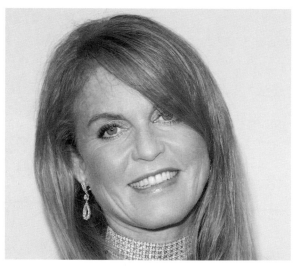

Sarah Ferguson's crowning glory has always been her fabulous red hair.

# Looking younger
## in your 40s

Women in their 40s should make the most of the colors that best complement their warm, glowing appearance. The emphasis here is on colors with a yellow-based undertone. Here's what will work for you.

## Warm colors you should use next to your face

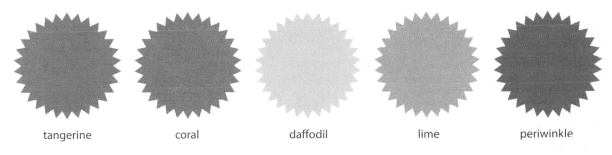

| tangerine | coral | daffodil | lime | periwinkle |

## Warm color combinations to try

| bittersweet | purple | mahogany | terracotta | evergreen |

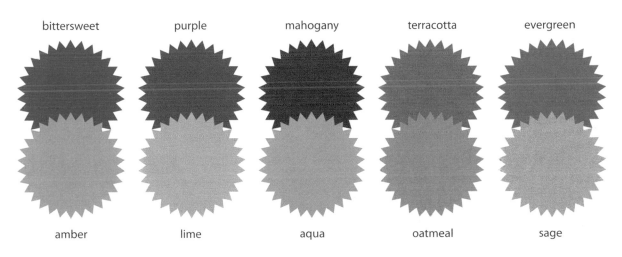

| amber | lime | aqua | oatmeal | sage |

# Looking younger
## in your 50s

For many women in their 50s this is the time to start using colors of a slightly softer shade near the face in order to avoid overwhelming their lighter skin tones and hair color.

## Warm colors you should use next to your face

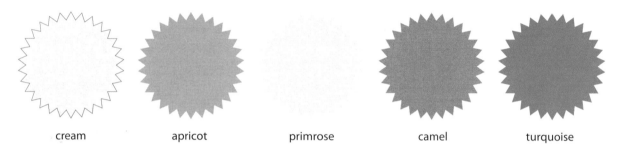

| cream | apricot | primrose | camel | turquoise |

## Light color combinations to try

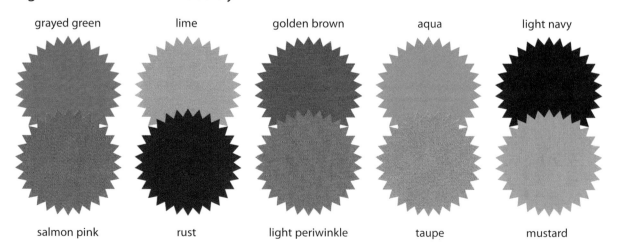

| grayed green | lime | golden brown | aqua | light navy |

| salmon pink | rust | light periwinkle | taupe | mustard |

# Looking younger
# in your 60s and beyond

Your coloring is now becoming fairly delicate, so avoid strong contrasting color combinations. Look for lighter, cooler versions of the colors you might have worn in your 40s and 50s (see pages 35–36).

## Warm colors you should use next to your face

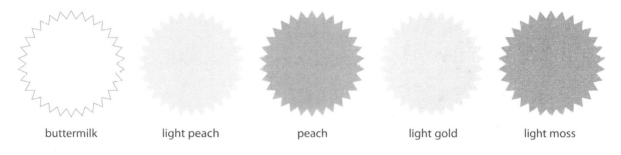

| buttermilk | light peach | peach | light gold | light moss |

## Warm color combinations to try

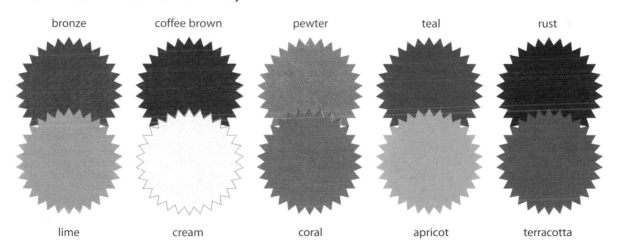

| bronze | coffee brown | pewter | teal | rust |
| lime | cream | coral | apricot | terracotta |

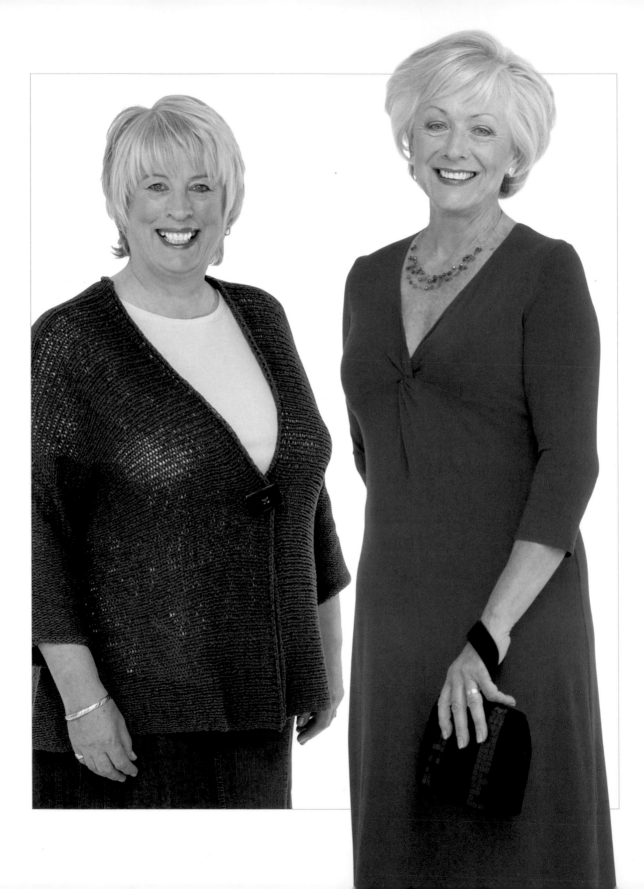

# Cool

If most or all of your color characteristics fall into this category, your overall appearance is likely to be cool and icy.

Your skin appears to have either pink undertones or, if you are dark-skinned, a slight blue tinge to it. There is not a hint of red in your hair; it's black, ash gray, silver-gray, or even pure white. The most important thing if your hair is gray is that you must have an up-to-date haircut to maintain a youthful look. Your eyes are blue, gray, or dark brown and may be soft and darkish or bright and sparkling.

## Key elements of your colors

There are a number of colors that you can wear well, referred to as your "palette" (see pages 40–41). When you assemble an outfit, however, always consider the following key elements.

### Depth: from light to medium

You need to balance the depth of your colors with the depth of your hair. The lighter your hair, the lighter the shades you should wear. Those of you with darker hair will be able to wear the darker tones of the palette, including black.

### Undertone: cool

All your colors need to have a cool (blue-based) undertone. Browns no longer complement your hair and skin; try pewter or charcoal instead.

### Clarity: clear or soft

If your eyes are bright you need some contrast in your look, either with brighter colors or makeup. Hot pink and medium gray are great. If your eyes are soft and dusky, try a more tonal look, like light periwinkle and purple.

## Accessories for a younger look

Don't underestimate the role accessories can play in your look. Hats, scarves, footwear, bags, and jewelry can all be used to give an outfit that extra style, while bringing your wardrobe staples right up to date. You can use them to break up simple lines, to accentuate your best features, and to add color or style without overpowering your look.

For shoes and bags, navy is the safest combination to wear with all your cool colors, and a pink handbag will add modernity to your look. Have some fun with colored shoes, too. With jewelry, go for silver, platinum, and white gold with rose quartz, sapphire, lapis, amethyst, or emerald. Your pearls should be pink, white or gray.

If you wear a scarf, choose brighter or lighter colors that will give you a natural face-lift.

Don't be afraid to use bold colors that contrast elegantly with your hair color.

# The cool palette

The colors listed here offer a good, basic range of what you should be looking for in order to stay looking young and radiant. Women in their 50s or 60s and beyond may find that their colors are lighter and cooler than in their 40s (see pages 43–45).

## Neutrals

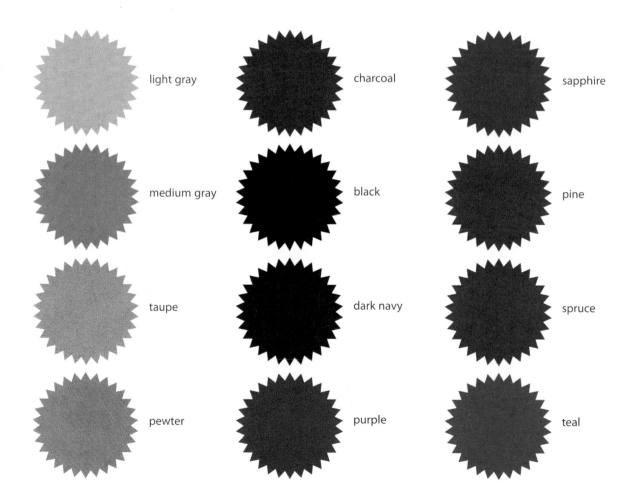

light gray

charcoal

sapphire

medium gray

black

pine

taupe

dark navy

spruce

pewter

purple

teal

## Lighter colors

soft white

rose beige

rose pink

baby pink

icy blue

icy green

## Fashion colors

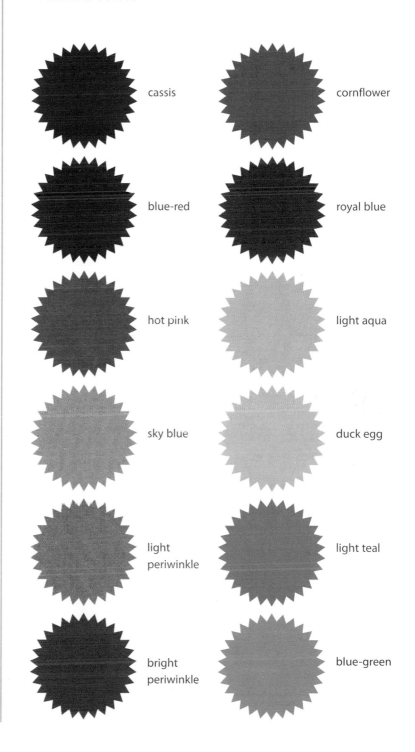

cassis

cornflower

blue-red

royal blue

hot pink

light aqua

sky blue

duck egg

light
periwinkle

light teal

bright
periwinkle

blue-green

# Looking younger with the **cool palette**

## Using your palette for a younger you

To achieve a youthful look with cool coloring you have to avoid wearing the "sweet pea" colors on their own. Although these colors can be very flattering, they need to be worn with some contrast or in an interesting outfit. If you have grayed prematurely don't be afraid to add color to your hair: ash tones or platinum blonde will complement your skin tones and eye color.

### The good news

As you continue to mature you will get cooler, so you can make those investment buys with confidence. Black is in your palette, but if you are in your late 50s and beyond, wear it with a low-cut neckline or in a lace or sheer fabric. A black-and-white woven fabric will give the illusion of being gray, which works incredibly well for you. Red is a great color with gray hair—go for it!

### The bad news

You need to be careful when wearing any beige or taupe pieces. These need to be accompanied by strong, cool colors. You also need to watch your eyebrows: make sure you remove any gray hairs or have them tinted regularly.

### The rules

- ✓ Ban anything with a yellow undertone from your closet or makeup bag.
- ✓ Contrast the darker shades of your palette with brighter or lighter colors.
- ✓ If you have a very high color to your face, use a skin adjuster to neutralize it.
- ✓ If your hair is light, replace black and navy with your blues and greens for a more youthful look.

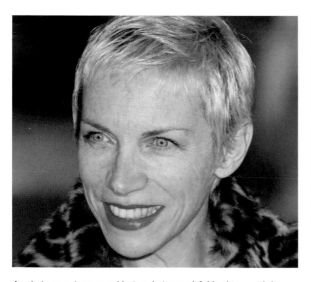

Annie Lennox's cropped hairstyle is youthful looking with her striking face.

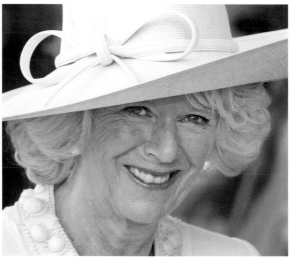

HRH The Duchess of Cornwall has matured beautifully in her palette of colors.

# Looking younger
## in your 40s

Women in their 40s will have no trouble wearing the more vibrant colors of the palette on pages 40–41 in order to keep looking young. Here's what will work for you.

## Cool colors you should use next to your face

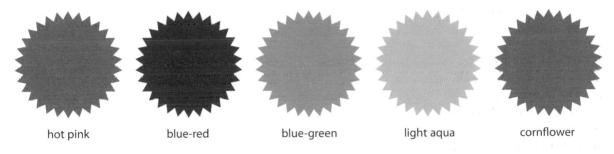

| hot pink | blue-red | blue-green | light aqua | cornflower |

## Cool color combinations to try

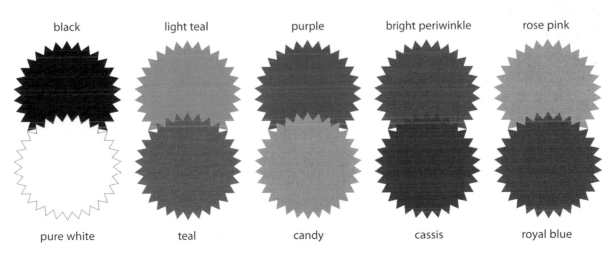

| black | light teal | purple | bright periwinkle | rose pink |
| pure white | teal | candy | cassis | royal blue |

# Looking younger
## in your 50s

Your natural coloring will be lighter now and will have lost a little contrast. Use the colors in your palette to energize your wardrobe and to achieve the contrast you may have lost.

## Cool colors you should use next to your face

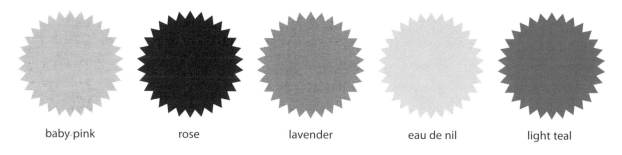

| baby pink | rose | lavender | eau de nil | light teal |

## Cool color combinations to try

| charcoal | denim | pine | periwinkle | cornflower |

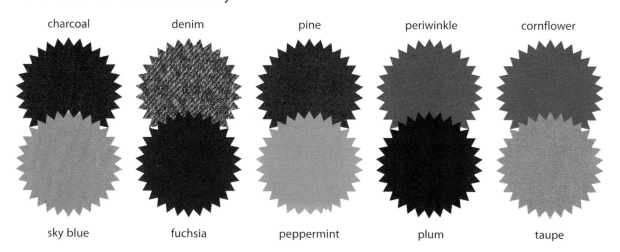

| sky blue | fuchsia | peppermint | plum | taupe |

# Looking younger
## in your 60s and beyond

Now that your coloring is becoming more delicate, you should avoid strong, contrasting color combinations. Go for lighter colors than you might have used in your 40s and 50s.

## Cool colors you should use next to your face

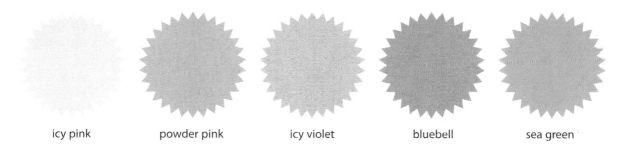

| icy pink | powder pink | icy violet | bluebell | sea green |

## Cool color combinations to try

| plum | blue-green | pewter | light gray | sapphire |

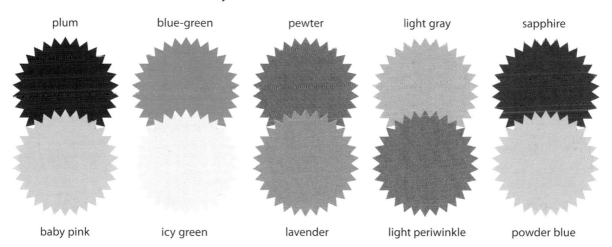

| baby pink | icy green | lavender | light periwinkle | powder blue |

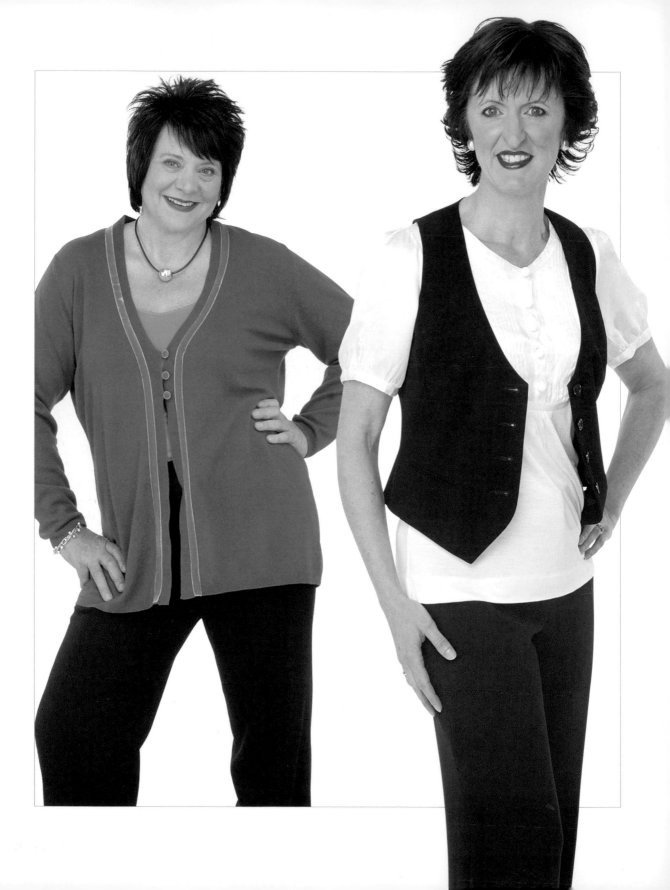

# Clear

If most or all of your color characteristics fall into this category, your overall appearance is likely to be both striking and bright.

Your look has always been dramatic, with your dark hair, clear and bright eyes, and clear complexion, whether your skin is porcelain or dark. Your eyebrows and eyelashes are dark. As long as you maintain the contrast between the darkness of your hair and the clarity of your eyes, your dominant will remain clear. The best colors for you are those that reflect that same brightness and contrast.

## Key elements of your colors

There are a number of colors that you can wear well, referred to as your "palette" (see pages 48–49). When you assemble an outfit, however, always consider the following key elements.

### Depth: from light to deep

The key to your look is contrast and you will do best by combining light and dark colors worn together. If you wear just one color, wear it near your face. The color must be bright, like emerald green or Chinese blue, for example.

### Undertone: warm or cool

If you have red, or warm, highlights to your hair (natural or otherwise), wear warmer (yellow-based) colors near your face, such as coral pink. Once you are graying, consider adding plum shades to your hair and wearing the cooler shades like candy near your face.

### Clarity: clear

All your colors are clear. When wearing your neutral colors, such as black or pewter, add contrasting color or bright accessories.

## Accessories for a younger look

Don't underestimate the role accessories can play in your look. Hats, scarves, footwear, bags, and jewelry can all be used to give an outfit that extra style, while bringing your wardrobe staples right up to date. Use them to break up simple lines, to accentuate your best features, and to add color or style without overpowering your look.

For shoes and bags, consider using black patent to complement your outfit instead of plain black, or any of your fashion colors. When it comes to jewelry, anything that sparkles will work for you; great stones and beads are emerald, sapphire, amethyst, ruby, and crystals.

Contrast between light and dark colors is a winning look for you. If you are just wearing one color, make sure it is a bright one.

# The clear palette

The colors listed here offer a good, basic range of what you should be looking for in order to stay looking young and radiant. Women in their 50s or 60s and beyond may find that their colors are lighter and cooler than in their 40s (see pages 51–53).

## Neutrals

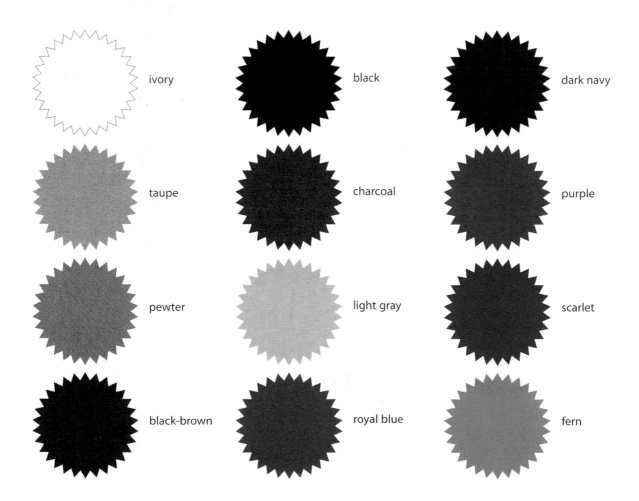

ivory

black

dark navy

taupe

charcoal

purple

pewter

light gray

scarlet

black-brown

royal blue

fern

## Lighter colors

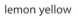

soft white

mint

lemon yellow

light apricot

light aqua

duck egg

## Fashion colors

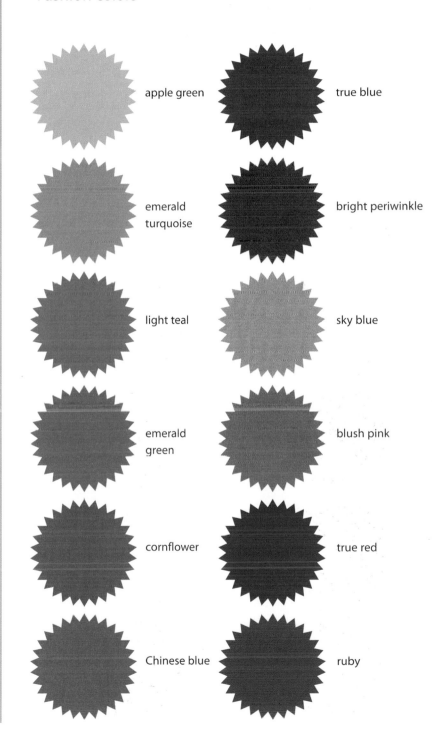

apple green

true blue

emerald turquoise

bright periwinkle

light teal

sky blue

emerald green

blush pink

cornflower

true red

Chinese blue

ruby

# Looking younger
## with the clear palette

## Using your palette for a younger you

You may be used to wearing black near your face (for example, in a turtleneck sweater) but now is the time to use black away from the face and to wear one of your beautiful, more striking colors here instead. Black and white will always work for you, but as the years pass, increase the percentage of white near the face. If and when your hair starts fading, consider enhancing the color to maintain the contrast.

### The good news

More than any of the other dominants, you can shop all year round because there are always colors from your palette in the stores. You can also have fun building up a colorful wardrobe of accessories that can be added to your neutrals anytime. Also, you are one of the few who can continue to look striking in black—as long as you add some bright colors to it.

### The bad news

Unfortunately, you do not look your best in beige, so you should avoid wearing it near your face if possible. If you wish to wear lighter colors in the summer, the best option is to add colors from your fashion palette in order to keep your look youthful. You have a tendency to go gray early, which means that you will need to consider tinting your hair.

### The rules

✓ Always wear contrasting or bright colors near your face.

✓ Don't wear dark colors on their own.

✓ Don't wear beiges and taupes on their own.

✓ Avoid wearing two pale colors near your face.

✓ Add contrasting-colored accessories.

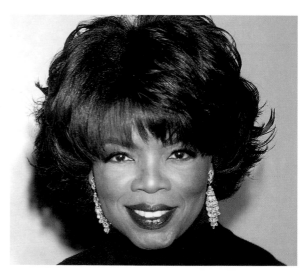

Liz Hurley's jewel-like eyes contrast beautifully with her hair and skin tone.

Oprah Winfrey's dark hair and clear, dark brown eyes are typical of a clear.

# Looking younger
## in your 40s

Of all the dominants, your natural coloring is best suited to wearing bright colors. Be bold enough to wear them with confidence, and you are guaranteed success time after time. Here's what works for you.

## Clear colors you should use next to your face

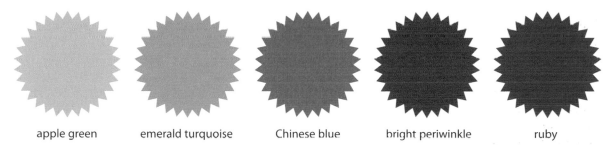

| apple green | emerald turquoise | Chinese blue | bright periwinkle | ruby |

## Clear color combinations to try

| charcoal | black-brown | denim | fern | blush pink |

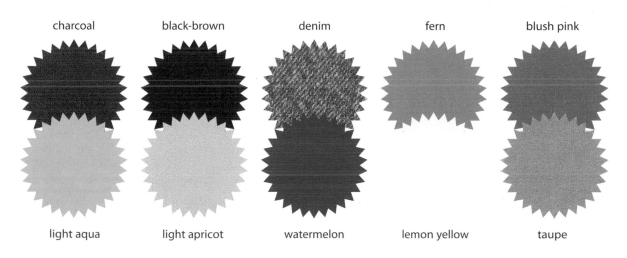

| light aqua | light apricot | watermelon | lemon yellow | taupe |

# Looking younger
## in your 50s

Women in their 50s may notice that their natural coloring is much lighter now. Remember that contrast is vital to your look— this may be the time to consider adding a tint to your hair to stay looking younger (see page 104).

## Clear colors you should use next to your face

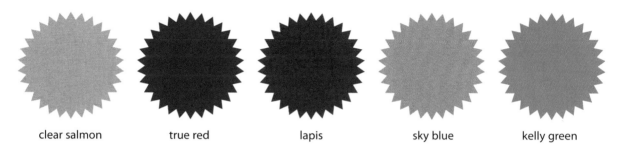

| clear salmon | true red | lapis | sky blue | kelly green |

## Clear color combinations to try

true blue | dark navy | ruby | pewter | light gray

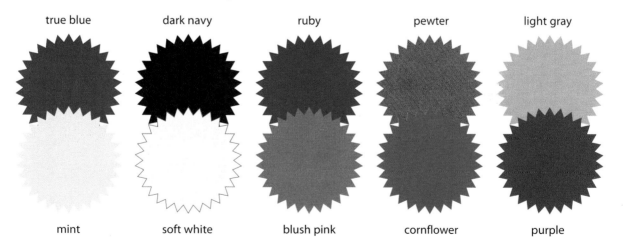

mint | soft white | blush pink | cornflower | purple

# Looking younger
## in your 60s and beyond

This is the time to assess your natural coloring and lighten the colors you might have worn in your 40s or 50s (see pages 51–52). In particular, you should start using cooler (blue-based) colors near your face.

## Clear colors you should use next to your face

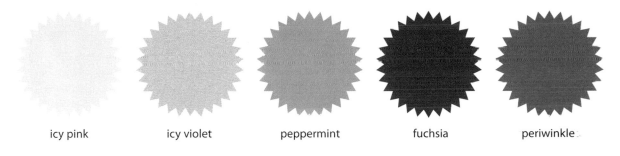

| icy pink | icy violet | peppermint | fuchsia | periwinkle |

## Clear color combinations to try

| powder blue | scarlet | dark teal | duck egg | violet |

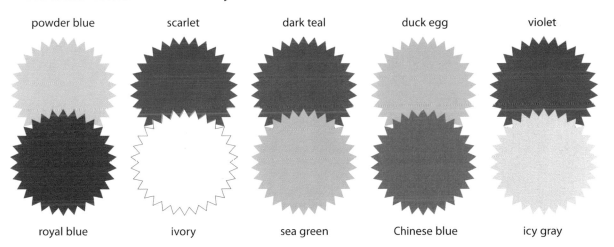

| royal blue | ivory | sea green | Chinese blue | icy gray |

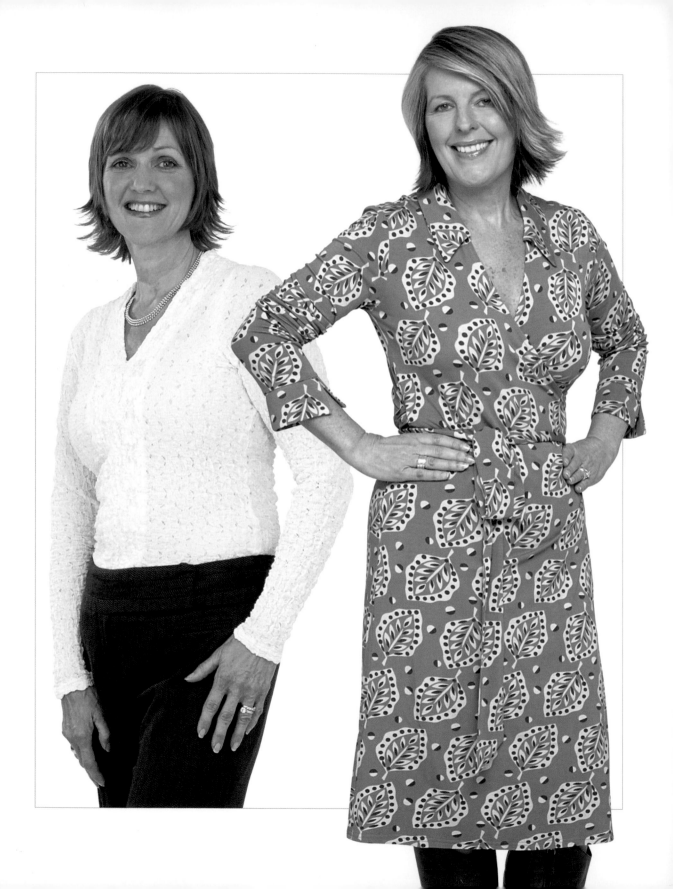

# Soft

If most or all of your color characteristics fall into this category, your overall appearance is likely to be muted and dusky.

You may have been blonde as a child, with your hair growing from dark blonde to medium brown. Your eye color is a combination of shades of greens, blues, and topaz brown. Your eyebrows and eyelashes will go from light to dark. Your skin tone is medium depth and you have an overall blended look with little contrast or definition. You don't have to worry as much as other dominant types now that you can see some grays coming through. These will just lift your natural color and appear as highlights in your hair, leaving you with the choice of going with the flow or adding a tint.

## Key elements of your colors
There are a number of colors that you can wear well, referred to as your "palette" (see pages 56–57). When you assemble an outfit, however, always consider the following key elements.

### Depth: medium
Your best shades are of medium depth like pewter or rose brown. Avoid wearing light colors on their own or, indeed, dark colors head to toe.

### Undertone: warm or cool
Both warm (yellow undertone) and cool (blue undertone) colors will work for you. If you have pink tones to your skin the cooler shades will be

more complementary near the face. If you have a slightly golden skin tone, the yellow-based colors will be best for you.

### Clarity: soft
All your colors need to be soft and muted. One way of achieving this is by using textured fabrics that absorb the light and therefore tone down the color. The use of tone-on-tone color is excellent (see pages 59–61).

## Accessories for a younger look
Don't underestimate the role accessories can play in your look. Hats, scarves, footwear, bags, and jewelry can all be used to give an outfit that extra style, while bringing your wardrobe staples right up to date. Use them to break up simple lines, to accentuate your best features, and to add color or style without overpowering your look.

Suede absorbs the brightness of a color and is therefore perfect for shoes and bags. When choosing jewelry, keep metals matte and the colors of your stones and beads either warm or cool: topaz, jade, amber, and tortoiseshell are warm; amethyst, opal, lapis, and rose quartz are cool. Pearls are perfect to mix together. Scarves in soft textures are also great.

Light neutrals are wonderful worn near the face, or go for subtle shades from your palette. Color combinations are blended rather than contrasting.

# The soft palette

The colors listed here offer a good, basic range of what you should be looking for in order to stay looking young and radiant. Women in their 50s or 60s and beyond may find that their colors are lighter and cooler than in their 40s (see pages 59–61).

## Neutrals

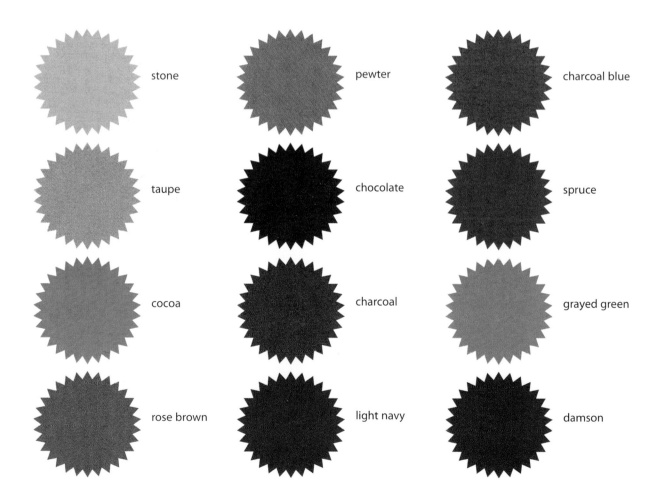

| | | |
|---|---|---|
| stone | pewter | charcoal blue |
| taupe | chocolate | spruce |
| cocoa | charcoal | grayed green |
| rose brown | light navy | damson |

# Lighter colors

soft white

shell

natural beige

mint

sage

sky blue

# Fashion colors

teal

jade

turquoise

emerald
turquoise

verbena

light
periwinkle

sapphire

soft violet

purple

blush pink

geranium

claret

# Looking younger
## with the **soft palette**

## Using your palette for a younger you

Your coloring will have cooled to varying degrees, depending on whether you have blue, green, or brown eyes. Replace warmer shades near your face with cooler ones—for example, verbena and sky blue. The darker shades in your palette should be worn with shades that are one or two tones lighter —for example, damson with soft violet, and chocolate with cocoa.

### The good news

Your colors are soft and blended, which means they will not overpower you and will be flattering near your face. The best news is that the neutral colors in your wardrobe will not have to change much over the years. You might just want to tweak the fashion colors from warm to cool in order to stay looking younger.

### The bad news

As your hair starts to gray more, shades like natural beige and shell will make your hair look yellow; it is best, therefore, to keep these shades to the bottom half of your body.

### The rules

✓ Wear medium-depth color.

✓ Blend colors together rather than wear clothes with high contrast.

✓ Lift the darker shades in your palette with colors one or two tones lighter.

✓ Choose accessories that tone with your outfit rather than contrast and stand out.

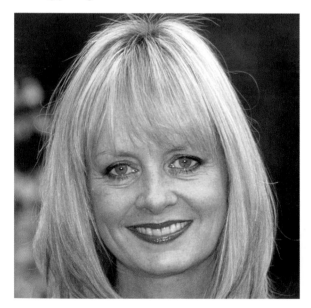

Twiggy's coloring has remained soft throughout her life, with her misty eyes and blonde hair.

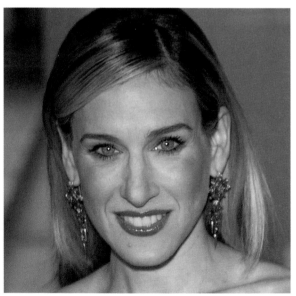

Sarah Jessica Parker's highlighted hair and soft green eyes make her a soft.

# Looking younger
## in your 40s

Many women in their 40s will find that their natural coloring is still very strong, and that they are therefore able to wear the bolder shades in their palette. Here's what will work for you.

## Soft colors you should use next to your face

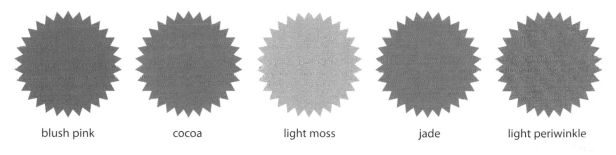

| blush pink | cocoa | light moss | jade | light periwinkle |

## Soft color combinations to try

| coffee brown | teal | sapphire | pewter | rust |

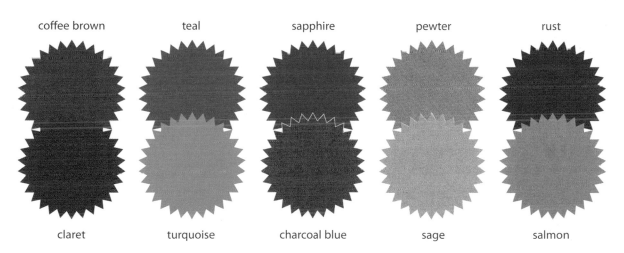

| claret | turquoise | charcoal blue | sage | salmon |

# Looking younger
## in your 50s

Your coloring is lighter and softer now. When choosing colors to wear near the face, look for shades in your palette that are a tone or two lighter than you might have worn in your 40s (see page 59).

## Soft colors you should use next to your face

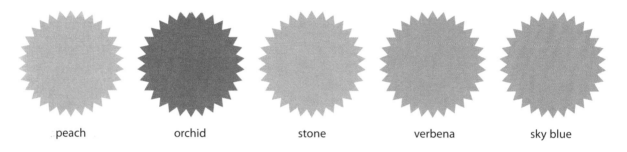

| peach | orchid | stone | verbena | sky blue |

## Soft color combinations to try

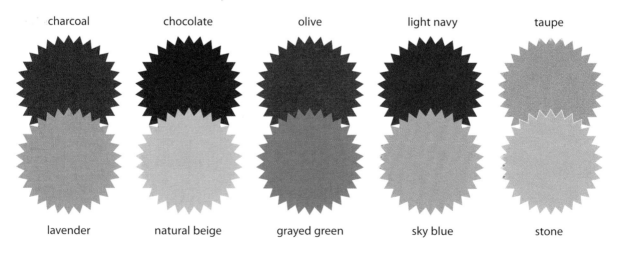

| charcoal | chocolate | olive | light navy | taupe |
| lavender | natural beige | grayed green | sky blue | stone |

# Looking younger
## in your 60s and beyond

Your natural coloring is probably a little cooler now than it was in your 40s and 50s (see pages 59–60), so try some of the blue-based colors in your palette.

## Soft colors you should use next to your face

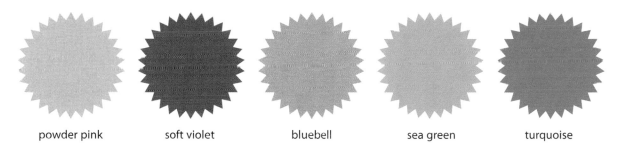

| powder pink | soft violet | bluebell | sea green | turquoise |

## Soft color combinations to try

| rose brown | spruce | purple | raspberry | emerald turquoise |

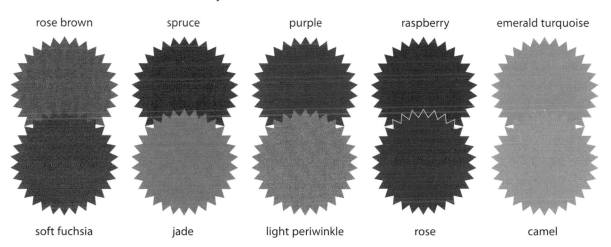

| soft fuchsia | jade | light periwinkle | rose | camel |

# A younger face

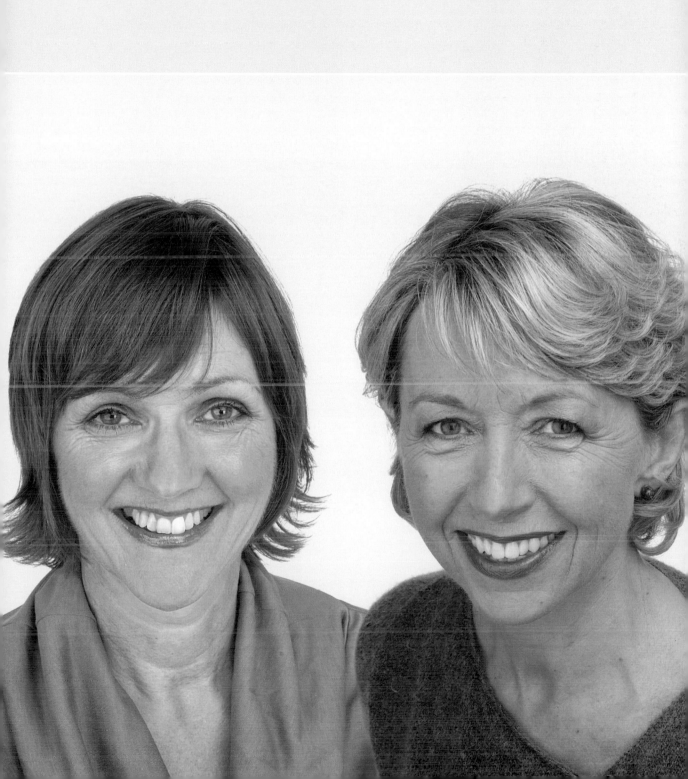

# Caring for your face

You cannot escape the signs of aging skin and loss of elasticity as you grow older: caused by a drop in natural estrogen in your system, it happens to everyone. Despite this, it is possible to adapt your daily beauty regime to stay younger looking for longer.

## Specialized skincare in the home

You may not be aware that your skin is the largest organ in your body and that, just like your heart, kidneys, or liver, it will get damaged if you abuse it. Properly cared for and maintained, however, your skin can remain perfectly healthy and in good condition to look youthful.

The key elements that damage your skin are sun, stress, smoking, diet, and airborne pollutants. Any medication you take may also have an effect on the appearance of your skin.

Over the last 20 years considerable progress has been made in developing a wide range of products that help protect the skin from these elements and slow down the aging process. Claims abound for products available over the counter (OTC), and it is right to say that the correct products for your skin type will help diminish the signs of aging and will give you a more youthful-looking skin.

## A good skincare routine

**Cleanse** Cleansers come as creams, lotions, and wash-off formulas. Generally, if your skin is still fairly oily, you may prefer to use a wash-off cleanser, moving on to a lotion or cream cleanser as your skin becomes drier.

**Tone** Always use a suitable toner for your skin type and ensure that all traces of your cleanser are removed. Any residue of the day's grime and makeup left on your face could cause blemishes and enlarged pores. Avoid astringents, which have an alcohol base that will dry the skin.

**Moisturize** Moisturizers are designed to protect the skin from the loss of natural moisture in the skin cells. You need to apply moisturizer every morning after cleansing and toning—even if you do not wear makeup—and don't forget your neck. Many moisturizers contain a sun protection factor, or SPF, but the majority do not give adequate protection. Experts say that the minimum SPF should be 30, whether you wear a foundation over it or not.

**Nourish** Nourishing creams penetrate into the deeper layers of the skin and help plump out the skin cells. Those of you in your 50s or 60s and beyond will need to use a richer nourishing cream as your skin dries and thins. Also, the addition of serums and balms will help improve your appearance and the visible signs of aging.

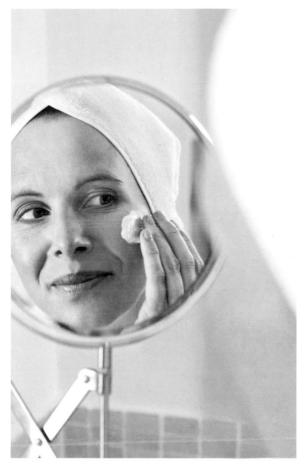
A twice-a-day skincare routine will guarantee a healthy skin, removing impurities and keeping it well nourished.

### Skin peels
These often contain alpha-hydroxy acids (AHAs), which help remove dead skin cells as you exfoliate. The AHAs also help diminish the look of fine lines and unclog pores. The process brings fresh, plumper cells to the surface, giving the skin a healthy-looking glow.

### Retinoids
A derivative of collagen-stimulating vitamin A, retinoids help renew the skin. At one time, they were only available by prescription. Today any OTC product containing even minute quantities of retinoids will definitely be more effective.

### Antioxidants
These include vitamins C and E, and are seen regularly in moisturizers and nourishing creams. They protect the skin from damaging free radicals (unstable molecules caused by pollution and other environmental factors), which cause visible signs of aging on the face and décolleté.

## Good skincare
There is no miracle cream for removing expression lines. Various treatments exist—from Botox injections to the full face-lift—but for the purposes of this book only noninvasive treatments are recommended.

If you are in your 40s and have never had a skincare routine, *now* is the time to start one. Regular application of moisturizing and nourishing creams will reduce the appearance of lines, whatever condition your skin is in—and that includes your neck and décolleté. It is not only the application of skin-care treatments that improves the skin condition, but also the twice-a-day gentle massaging that helps improve the circulation.

### Eye creams and gels
The skin around the eyes is different from the rest of the face and needs specialized creams. A lightweight gel applied under your eye makeup is perfect for the day; a richer cream will hydrate the skin while you sleep.

### Face masks
These come in various forms. Those with a clay base tend to dry on the surface of the skin, removing impurities, sloughing off dead skin cells, and minimizing enlarged pores. Glycerin-based masks, which remain soft on the face, are intended to soften and hydrate the skin. Your face will feel refreshed and properly cleansed.

# Makeup

Wearing great makeup is one of the easiest ways of maintaining your youthful looks, primarily because it evens out the telltale signs of aging. Find out which products work best for you and learn how to apply them well.

The basis of any good makeup is starting with a perfect canvas. This becomes increasingly difficult with age, but with the clever use of skin primers and a good-quality foundation, it can be achieved with little effort. All makeup should be applied to a clean, toned, and moisturized face (see page 64).

## The tools
- Cosmetic sponges
- Concealer brush
- Sponge-tipped applicator
- Powder puff
- Cotton pad
- Powder brush

### Power surges

Also known as "hot flashes," power surges generally occur in women going through the menopause, when estrogen is low. They may be frequent at night, when they become "night sweats" and may make it difficult to get a good night's sleep. If you have a power surge you will experience a feeling of intense heat with sweating that may last for up to 30 minutes. They may happen a few times a week or constantly throughout the day.

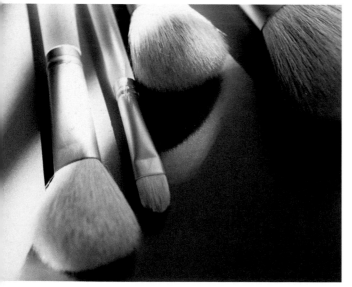

## The products
There are a number of products you can use to help you achieve a youthful appearance.

### Skin primer/adjuster
These come in different colors. Yellow blends any uneven pigmentation or discoloration of the skin and green helps camouflage high color caused by broken capillaries. This is very helpful if you suffer from "power surges." Lavender skin primer will warm up a yellow or sallow skin tone.
**Application:** Either using a cosmetic sponge or your fingertips, apply the appropriate skin adjuster lightly over the offending area.

Using good brushes will make your makeup application easier and more professional.

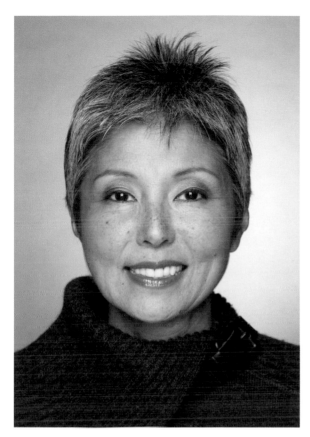

A perfectly applied foundation gives the perfect canvas for makeup application.

## Foundation

Your choice of foundation will depend on personal preference, climate, and lifestyle. Choosing the color is the main issue here. Foundation should not "sit" visibly on the face, but should blend in with your natural coloring at the jawline. To choose the right color for you, apply a small amount to the side of your face—not the back of your hand. It should just blend in and look natural.
**Application:** Apply with a cosmetic sponge for an allover, even finish. Start on either cheek, gently patting and stippling, and continue to work around the face, avoiding eyelids and lips. Lightly blend out toward the hair- and jawlines, avoiding any visible lines. Do not start by dabbing dots of foundation all over your face: these products are designed to dry on contact with the air and if you use this method they will dry unevenly.

## Concealer

This is essential, whatever your age! Concealer has a fairly dense formulation and is best applied on top of foundation. Some have light-diffusing properties, which are excellent for camouflaging blemishes and dark circles under the eyes.
**Application:** Apply with a sponge-tipped applicator or a small concealer brush, then blend into the foundation gently with your fingertip.

## Loose powder

For a long-lasting and professional look, loose powder is a must-have product. It helps set the foundation, thus keeping your face fresh-looking all day. Keep shine under control with a little powder. A translucent shade is the best and easiest to use.
**Application:** Apply either with a clean powder puff or a cotton pad by rolling it gently onto the face, avoiding the eye area. Then, using a powder brush, brush off excess powder with downward strokes to smooth down facial down/hair.

### Tips

**In your 40s:** Now is the time to give up your tinted moisturizer and to start using foundation and powder. Don't forget your concealer for camouflaging the odd blemish that might still appear.

**In your 50s:** Use powder just on the bony part of your face —powder gathered in your expression lines will only emphasize them. Apply concealer to the innermost corner of the eye for a more youthful look.

**In your 60s and beyond:** Once you start losing some of your natural coloring, your skin may benefit from a lavender skin adjuster. Apply concealer to the deepest lines on your face to help lessen their appearance. Blend it well.

# Making up your eyes

Your eyes are a vital communication tool, and eye makeup helps draw attention to them, particularly if you have a pale complexion. Making up your eyes properly is one of the most important stages of grooming.

## The tools
- Pencil sharpener
- Cotton swabs
- Blender brush
- Angled eye shadow brush
- Tweezers
- Eyebrow brush
- Eyelash curlers (optional)

## The products
Whether you are in your 40s, 50s, or 60s and beyond you will use the same products, but the way you apply them or the shades you use may change.

### Eye base
This is a specially formulated product designed to hold eye shadow in place, and can also prevent deeper shades of eye shadow staining the fine, delicate skin of the eyelid.
**Application:** Apply evenly over the entire eyelid from lashes to brow with your index figure.

### Eye pencils
Kinder on the eyelid than a liquid eyeliner, these are also more youthful looking. Choose a shade to suit your dominant coloring palette.
**Application:** Always sharpen before use. Starting at the outer edge of the upper lid, gently apply as close to the lashes as possible, approximately two-thirds of the way along. For the lower lid, apply close to the lashes, starting at the outer edge to halfway along. Soften the lines with a cotton swab.

## The eyebrows

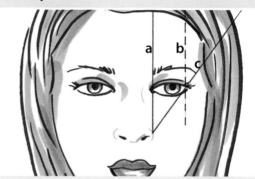

The perfect frame for any eye shape is a well-groomed eyebrow. You can give yourself an instant face-lift by reshaping your brows using the following steps:

- Pluck away any stray hairs between the brows.

- Make sure the inner corner of the brow lines up with the inner corner of the eye.

- Remove any long or graying hairs with tweezers, pulling in the direction of the hair growth.

- Enhance the natural arch by removing stray hairs from underneath.

- If necessary, lengthen and fill in brows with a brown pencil to match hair/eyebrow color.

- Make sure the natural length extends beyond the outer edge of the eye.

# Tips

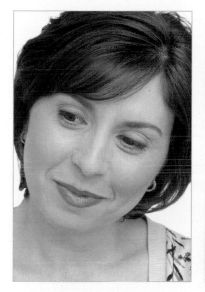

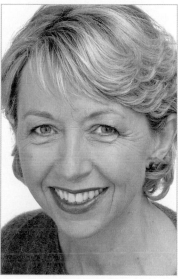

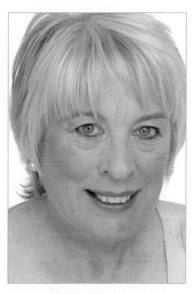

**In your 40s:** Abandon frosted eye shadows, which will only emphasize crepiness on the eyelid. Don't be afraid to experiment with eye shadow colors and combinations.

**In your 50s:** Use eye base to make sure your eye shadow doesn't crease during the day. If your eyebrows and lashes start to fade, consider having them professionally tinted.

**In your 60s and beyond:** To help lift the outer corner of your eye, apply more eye pencil to the lower lid than on the top. Abandon mascara on the lower lashes—the idea is to revert to a more natural look as you age.

## Eye shadow

Powder eye shadows are much easier to use than cream ones, the latter being harder to blend and tending to crease. Choose at least two shades of complementing colors from your palette. Matte and shimmering eye shadows are far more flattering and youthful looking.

**Application:** Gently lift the eyelid upward, holding the brow (this will flatten any crepiness on the eyelid, where the skin becomes stretched and falls into loose folds). Use a blender brush to apply a base color all over the entire eyelid. Apply other colors to suit your eye shape, using an angled brush. Blend all colors together with the blender brush.

## Mascara

Available in many colors and formulations, be sure to choose one that not only complements your natural coloring, but also does not overload your lashes with heavy fibers. The most flattering colors are black, brown and navy—at all costs avoid bright fashion colors. Make sure you replace your mascara regularly (every three months at the most) to avoid eye infections.

**Application:** Gently turn the mascara wand in the tube (pumping forces air into the tube, which dries the mascara prematurely). By wiping the mascara wand over the top of the eyelashes you will remove any excess eye shadow, while adding volume to your lashes.

# Blushers, bronzers, and highlighters

Applying these products will help contour your face and shape it in a flattering, natural way. A dash of blusher swept over the cheekbones will always make you look younger and healthier.

## The tools
• Blush brush

## The products
To achieve a younger and healthy look there are three different products you can use.

### Blusher
There are cream and powder blushers. Choose a color that complements your dominant palette.

**Application:** You apply cream blusher directly to the face or on top of your foundation before powdering. Gently pat along the cheekbones with the fingertips, blending the blusher in gently. You can apply powder directly to the skin or on top of powder with a blush brush. For the best effect, whether using cream or powder, apply it to the top of the cheekbones upward and toward the hairline. Make sure it does not come too far forward to the front of your face.

### Bronzing powder
Over the years bronzing powders have become more and more popular as women have realized that although a tan gives you a wonderful healthy glow, it is better to apply it artificially. Bronzers are generally used more in the summer than in the winter.

**Application:** Using a blush brush, apply the powder lightly over the area of the face that would naturally be hit by the sun. Don't forget your neck and shoulders if you are wearing a strappy top. You can apply this either straight onto the face or over your foundation and powder.

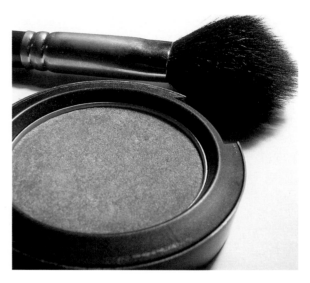

A blush powder or bronzer is great for an instant face-lift—it helps contour your face and provide a healthy glow.

### Highlighter
This comes in cream or powder formulations, and is used in conjunction with blusher and bronzer. The rule is that if you shade an area on the face you need to highlight it as well. Choose a highlighter that shimmers rather than glitters. Natural shimmers add light and contour to a face that could be losing definition.

Highlighters can be used to define and draw attention to any area on your face. This is particularly useful when you have a slight tan on your face.

**Application:** Apply powder with a blush brush and cream with your fingertips. On all faces, apply a touch of shimmer around the outer eye area and upper cheekbones.

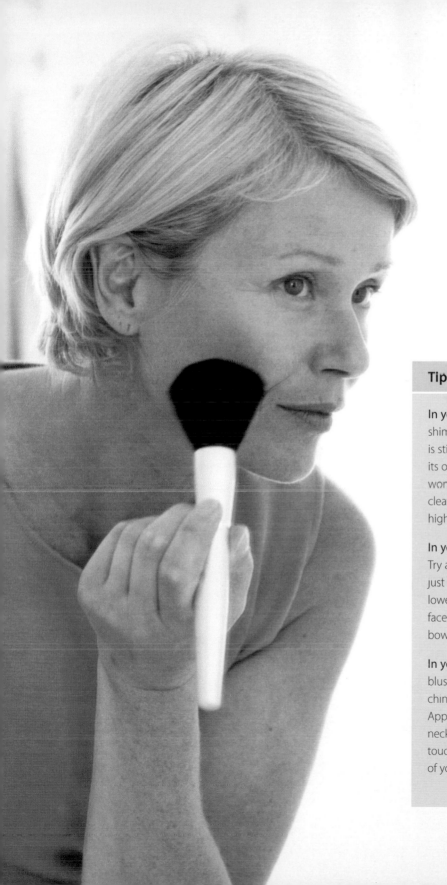

## Tips

**In your 40s:** Try choosing a blusher with a little shimmer for your evening look (your skin is still good and line free). Use the bronzer on its own—that is, without foundation—for a wonderfully natural look. To accentuate your cleavage, use a bronzer in the center and the highlighter on either side.

**In your 50s:** Stick to matte shades of blusher. Try a lighter one on top with a deeper shade just below it. Use the bronzer lightly along the lower jawbone to give added definition to your face. Dab a little highlighter over the Cupid's bow to lift the upper lip for a fuller smile.

**In your 60s and beyond:** After applying blusher to your cheekbones, add a dab to your chin and nose to give yourself a healthy glow. Apply lightly underneath the chin and on the neck to help camouflage a double chin. Add a touch of highlighter underneath the outer edge of your eyebrows to lift the eyes.

# Making up your lips

A significant sign of aging is loss of color from the lips—gone are the days when you can simply get away with a light lip gloss. You should now be looking to give your lips a fresh burst of life.

In your 40s, your lips begin to lose color and the teenage pout disappears. In your 50s and beyond, your lips will thin (because of the decrease of collagen production) and fine lines will appear around them. If you have smoked, these lines will begin to appear a lot earlier.

## The tools
- Pencil sharpener
- Lip brush
- Tissues

## The products
Following are the products you can use to give shape to your lips, to help ensure that your lipstick or lip gloss stay on longer and to provide that final professional touch to your makeup.

### Lip base
Applied over your lips before adding color, a lip base will not only moisturize your lips, but will ensure that the color stays true, giving a long-lasting finish.
**Application:** Using its applicator, apply evenly all over your lips. Smile gently as you do so to make sure the base gets into the fine lines on your lips.

### Lip pencils
Lip pencils give depth to the lipstick and gloss color, definition to the lip line, and also help to stop your lipstick from "bleeding." You should have a range of different color pencils to complement and enhance your lipsticks and glosses.

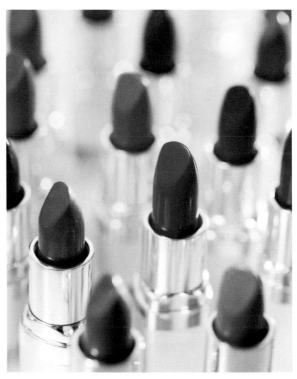

Have a selection of different shades of lipsticks to suit your mood and the occasion.

**Application:** Apply to the outer edge of the lips, starting at the middle and following the natural lip line. Fill in to give a base color to your lipstick or gloss. Avoid applying a dark color just to outline your lips: this is very aging, especially when your lipstick wears off.

### Lipsticks
There are many formulations of lipstick available, from cream to sheer. Choose colors that

complement your natural coloring. Lipstick is one of the first things other people notice about you, so it is important to get it right.

**Application:** For a long-lasting look, apply with a lip brush. Work the brush into the lipstick, then apply evenly all over the lips (still smiling). Blot with tissues and reapply.

## Lip gloss

This can be used on its own, in conjunction with a lip pencil, or over a lipstick. Used all over the lips, or at the middle of the upper lip, a gloss will give you the appearance of a fuller mouth.

**Application:** Apply with its own applicator or a lip brush.

## Lip fixers

These products are designed to seal the color onto the lips.

**Application:** Apply following the manufacturer's instructions and leave to dry properly before eating or drinking.

## Tips

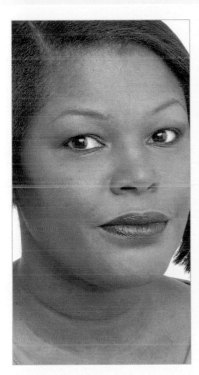

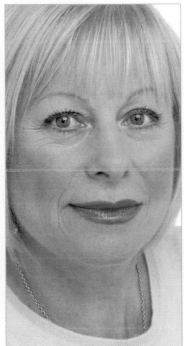

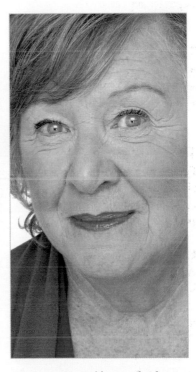

**In your 40s:** Have fun layering lip pencil, lipstick, and gloss to create interesting combinations of color.

**In your 50s:** Get rid of any frosted lipsticks you may still have. Go for sheer or cream formulations. Add gloss for a touch of glamour.

**In your 60s and beyond:** After applying lipstick, reapply your lip pencil to the outer edge of your lips for greater definition.

# The natural face-lift

It is not necessary to resort to surgery to correct the signs of aging. By using a combination of light (to emphasize) and dark (to minimize) it is amazing how you can create the illusion of a perfect face.

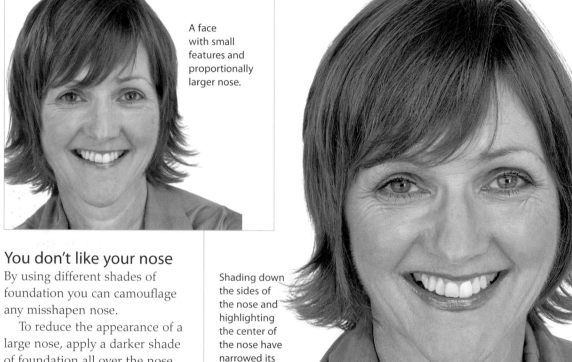

A face with small features and proportionally larger nose.

Shading down the sides of the nose and highlighting the center of the nose have narrowed its appearance.

## You don't like your nose

By using different shades of foundation you can camouflage any misshapen nose.

To reduce the appearance of a large nose, apply a darker shade of foundation all over the nose and use a highlighter along the top of your cheekbone. Choose a hairstyle that allows you to have some volume.

To reduce the width of a flat nose, apply a darker foundation on either side of the nose and use a highlighter down the center of the nose.

## You need to build up your chin

Some women lose the definition of a firm chin either through a loss of tightness of facial tissue or by gaining a little weight. It is not necessary to resort to implants to regain your chin.

Apply a highlighter to the chin area, while using a darker powder underneath the chin. This will draw attention to the chin, making it appear pert and firmer.

## You want to get rid of those chins

Liposuction and tucks should be a last resort. Clever use of powders and some tricks of the trade will help make your double chin disappear.

Use a darker shade of face powder underneath the jaw and down the neck. This will give the illusion of a natural shadow, reducing the appearance of your chin(s). Draw attention to either your eyes or your lips by using more color, and avoid high necklines, tight scarves, and very short necklaces that finish near your chin(s).

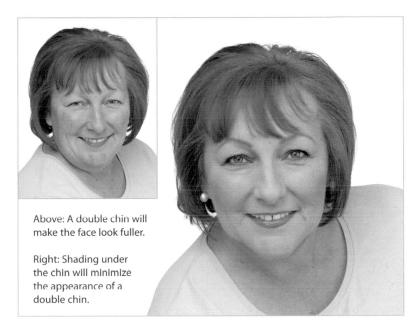

Above: A double chin will make the face look fuller.

Right: Shading under the chin will minimize the appearance of a double chin.

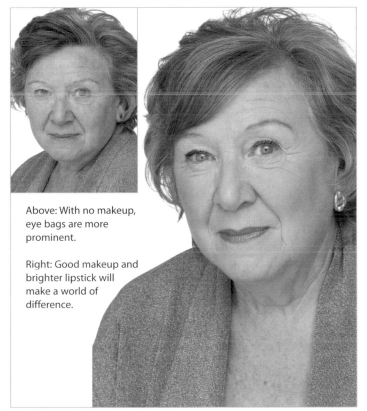

Above: With no makeup, eye bags are more prominent.

Right: Good makeup and brighter lipstick will make a world of difference.

## You have bags under your eyes

There are many different causes for bags and circles under the eyes: lack of sleep, a bad diet, a cold, stress, and the general aging process among them. To start with, you could improve your diet and drink plenty of water.

The easiest way to disguise dark circles and bags with makeup is to apply a concealer or yellow-based skin primer over the offending area before applying foundation. Use a brush and make sure the concealer is light in texture (you don't want to pull the delicate skin).

If the bags are puffy make sure you are not using too rich a cream near your eyes (or too much of it). Use a colored eyeliner on the top lid of the eye to detract attention from the lower eye area. Using lots of mascara on the upper lashes will also help. Wearing as bright a lipstick as your palette allows will take attention away from your eyes. Earrings will distract onlookers, too.

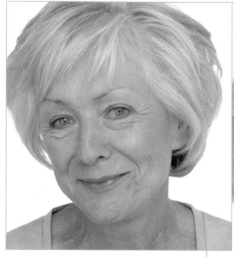
The eyes are lost without definition.

## You have thinning eyelashes and faint brows

As you age, you may find your hair getting thinner. For some women this could include eyebrows and lashes.

Consider having your eyebrows tinted professionally, or use a colored pencil to fill in. Avoid any temptation to have your eyebrows permanently tattooed. Although it might be effective at first, your eyebrows will become a mess of lines as you age.

To build up your eyelashes, apply several coats of mascara, letting it dry between coats. If your lashes are light in color, you could consider tinting them.

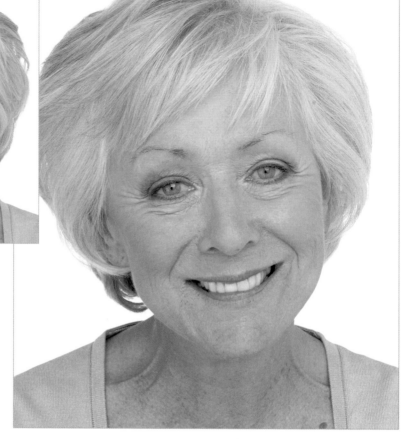
Eyebrows are the picture frame for your eyes, enhancing your total look.

## You have a droopy or hooded eyelid

This is when the flesh of the upper part of the eye falls in a fold over the eyelid, covering it. By using light and dark eye shadows, you can enhance the appearance of the eye.

Apply eye base all over the eye, lifting the brow to ensure even distribution, then apply a light-colored eye shadow all over the eye area. Draw your eye pencil two-thirds of the way along below the eye, from the outside corner inward. Using an angled or contour brush, and a neutral color such as a medium brown, apply the shadow in an arch on the fleshy part of the skin that hangs over the lid. The effect is to minimize the expanse of skin. Apply a light shade of eye shadow on the lid near the lashes; this will bring the lid forward. Apply more mascara to the outer edges to lift the eye.

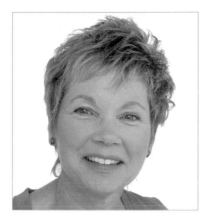

Above: Eyes look small with little or no makeup.

Right: Clever application of eye shadow in the right place enhances the eyes.

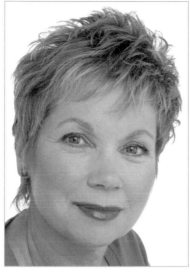

## You have deep-set eyes

As the muscles around the eyes age they can slacken, leaving the eyes set deeper in the skull. A professional secret here is to keep the color of the eye shadows light.

Apply eye base, and then a light color all over the eye area. Draw a fine line along the edge of the upper lid with your pencil and halfway along underneath. Use a bright apricot/pink color right in the socket of the eye to bring it forward. Apply mascara evenly all over.

## You have feathering lips

This is where fine lines appear around the edge of the mouth, mainly caused by smoking, although genetics plays its part. The skin on your lips, like that of your eyes, is very thin and has very few oil glands, which is why these areas age first. Use a small amount of your eye cream or gel around the mouth and the lips to moisturize and nourish.

Apply lip base all over and be sure to give a firm pencil outline to your lips before and after applying color. Be careful when using very soft lip gloss or a very dark color as these tend to bleed into the fine lines.

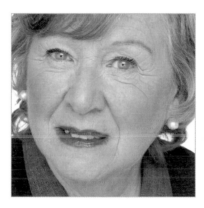

Above: Lipstick bleeding into the teathering of the lips looks aging.

Right: Careful application of lipstick and lip pencil will camouflage feathering around the lips.

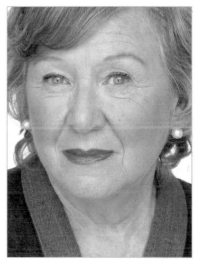

## You have thinning lips

Avoid the temptation to have collagen injections, which can result in ugly, pouting lips. Instead, use color to give the appearance of a fuller mouth.

Start by applying lip base all over. Then, using a natural pale pink or peach pencil, apply lip pencil just on the outer edge of your lip line and fill in. Use the lightest color of lipstick from your palette before applying lip gloss just to the center of the lips to plump up.

# Disguising signs of age with makeup

Don't panic over the normal aging of your skin. The process is inevitable and is caused both by your lifestyle and your genes. There are a number of ways you can lessen its appearance.

## Lines and wrinkles

These are your awards for having laughed and cried! Aging, of course, owes much to exposure to light, wind, sun, and artificial heating. A good skin-care routine, started at an early age, will slow down the appearance of lines and wrinkles (see page 64).

A light touch to your makeup and its application will ensure that the lines and wrinkles are not emphasized. For this reason, you should avoid heavy concealers, foundations, and powders, which will only build up in your lines.

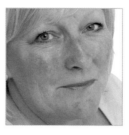

Broken capillaries can easily be disguised by using skin primer under your foundation.

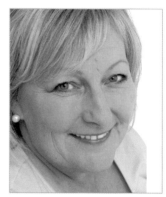

A naked face shows all the signs of lines and wrinkles.

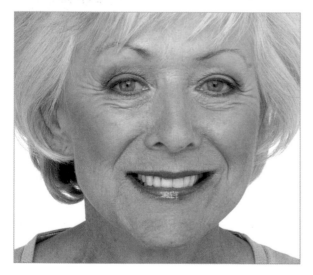

Well-applied makeup enhances the eyes and smile for a younger look.

## Broken capillaries

These fine red lines can appear anywhere on the face, and can be aggravated by stimulants in your diet such as coffee and alcohol. They also tend to manifest themselves at the time of the menopause. Using a green-based skin primer underneath your foundation will help camouflage them.

## Skin tags and facial warts

These can appear anywhere on the face and neck and, if they are small, you can disguise them with concealer. You can also have them easily removed professionally.

## Age spots

These are areas of dark pigmentation of the skin that develop more with exposure to daylight—the more exposure, the darker the spots. Sun filters and blocks are a must. Don't try to camouflage age spots on your face with heavy foundation; a yellow-based skin primer will help minimize their effect.

**Facial hair** Hormonal changes may result in the appearance of coarse facial hair. There are various methods of removal, including electrolysis, laser, and waxing. An expert will advise on the best method of removal for you.

**Facials** Nothing is more relaxing than a facial—just make sure you schedule it for a time when you can keep on relaxing afterward. The skin is stimulated and will continue to respond long after the treatment is over, so no makeup either. A facial can be anything from relaxing to intensive. Your beautician will establish your skin type and needs while inquiring about your skincare routine.

This is a great way to revitalize and restore the skin's natural radiance and vitality after exposure to pollution and environmental aggressors (air conditioning, indoor heating). A gentle and stimulating facial massage will boost the blood circulation (expect to leave the cubicle looking a little red in the face). The delicate eye area is targeted to soothe away fine lines and wrinkles, while dark circles and puffiness are reduced. Hydrating your skin will be part of the treatment.

**Dental care** Regular visits to your dentist and hygienist are an essential part of looking after your smile. The state of your teeth in your 40s, 50s, 60s, and beyond will largely depend on the care and maintenance you had in previous decades. Investing in crowns, veneers, and even orthodontistry can be money well spent.

There are many products available over the counter for bleaching and whitening teeth. Your dentist is the expert and you should take his advice before starting any regime.

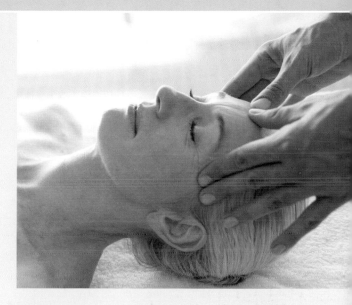

**Eyebrow shaping** If you overplucked your eyebrows in your younger days, or if the hairs are growing long and out of shape, you may want to get expert help to reshape them. Professionals will use wax, tweezers, or threading—or even a combination of all three—to create the perfect brow. Beware of using scissors, as they blunt the end of the hair and make brows look coarse.

**Eyebrow tinting** Just like your hair, your brows may need some tinting to give your eyebrows some definition and shape, particularly if you are blonde or have gone gray. Make sure you don't go too dark; the color must look natural.

**Eyelash dye** Lashes can be colored using a natural vegetable dye, and there is a range of colors to choose from, although blondes must be careful not to go too dark. The treatment should last at least six weeks.

# Makeup for the
# light dominant

Whether you are in your 40s, 50s, or 60s and beyond, your primary aim with makeup is to keep all your colors and their application light and delicate in order to harmonize with your natural coloring.

## Combinations

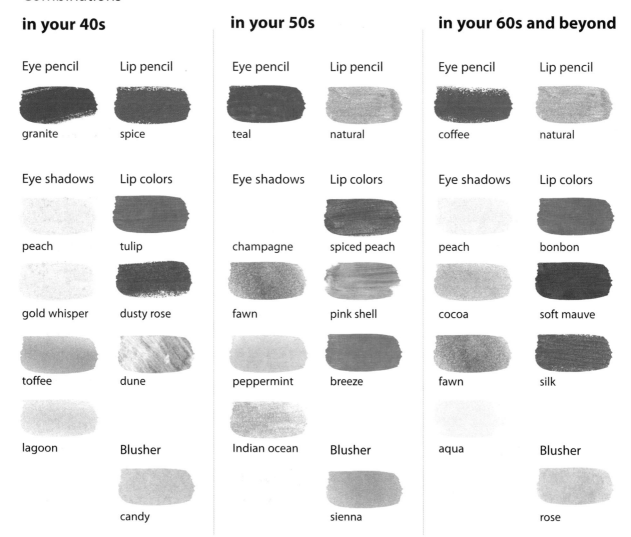

### in your 40s

| Eye pencil | Lip pencil |
|---|---|
| granite | spice |

| Eye shadows | Lip colors |
|---|---|
| peach | tulip |
| gold whisper | dusty rose |
| toffee | dune |
| lagoon | Blusher |
| | candy |

### in your 50s

| Eye pencil | Lip pencil |
|---|---|
| teal | natural |

| Eye shadows | Lip colors |
|---|---|
| | champagne |
| fawn | spiced peach |
| peppermint | pink shell |
| Indian ocean | breeze |
| | Blusher |
| | sienna |

### in your 60s and beyond

| Eye pencil | Lip pencil |
|---|---|
| coffee | natural |

| Eye shadows | Lip colors |
|---|---|
| peach | bonbon |
| cocoa | soft mauve |
| fawn | silk |
| aqua | Blusher |
| | rose |

# Makeup for the
## deep dominant

Dark, strong colors will balance with your look in your 40s, but expect to lighten up, both in terms of color and application, if you are in your 50s or 60s and beyond.

## Combinations

### in your 40s

| Eye pencil | Lip pencil |
|---|---|
| aubergine | russet |

| Eye shadows | Lip colors |
|---|---|
| melon | tomato |
| mocha | ruby |
| lavender bliss | sangria |
| mercury | Blusher |
| | marsala |

### in your 50s

| Eye pencil | Lip pencil |
|---|---|
| olive | red |

| Eye shadows | Lip colors |
|---|---|
| apricot | pecan |
| cocoa | savannah |
| steel | kazzbar |
| smoke | Blusher |
| | port |

### in your 60s and beyond

| Eye pencil | Lip pencil |
|---|---|
| brown | natural |

| Eye shadows | Lip colors |
|---|---|
| peach | nutmeg |
| fawn | ruby |
| khaki | mahogany |
| apricot | Blusher |
| | candy |

# Makeup for the
# warm dominant

It is important for you to remember to keep the undertone of your makeup colors warm, whatever your age. Even when a few gray hairs appear, avoid the cool pink shades of lipstick.

## Combinations

### in your 40s

| Eye pencil | Lip pencil |
|---|---|
| moss | cantaloupe |

| Eye shadows | Lip colors |
|---|---|
| apricot | copper |
| cocoa | tangerine |
| khaki | sunset |
| Indian ocean | Blusher |
| | cognac |

### in your 50s

| Eye pencil | Lip pencil |
|---|---|
| brown | russet |

| Eye shadows | Lip colors |
|---|---|
| melon | terracotta |
| mocha | nutmeg |
| smoke | warm sand |
| gold whisper | Blusher |
| | almond |

### in your 60s and beyond

| Eye pencil | Lip pencil |
|---|---|
| coffee | spice |

| Eye shadows | Lip colors |
|---|---|
| peach | topaz |
| fawn | coral |
| grayed green | rum |
| tangerine | Blusher |
| | muscat |

# Makeup for the
## cool dominant

Whether you are in your 40s, 50s, or 60s and beyond, the key to your look is keeping your colors cool. Brighten your lipstick if you have lost all the color from your hair and are now white.

## Combinations

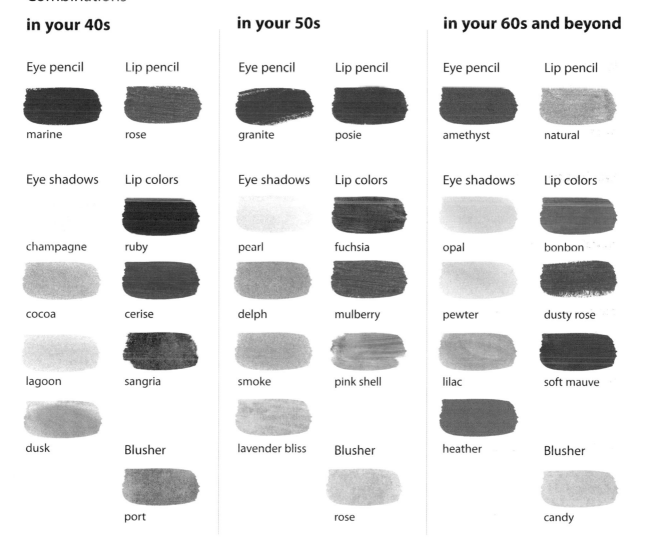

### in your 40s

| Eye pencil | Lip pencil |
|---|---|
| marine | rose |

| Eye shadows | Lip colors |
|---|---|
| champagne | ruby |
| cocoa | cerise |
| lagoon | sangria |
| dusk | Blusher |
| | port |

### in your 50s

| Eye pencil | Lip pencil |
|---|---|
| granite | posie |

| Eye shadows | Lip colors |
|---|---|
| pearl | fuchsia |
| delph | mulberry |
| smoke | pink shell |
| lavender bliss | Blusher |
| | rose |

### in your 60s and beyond

| Eye pencil | Lip pencil |
|---|---|
| amethyst | natural |

| Eye shadows | Lip colors |
|---|---|
| opal | bonbon |
| pewter | dusty rose |
| lilac | soft mauve |
| heather | Blusher |
| | candy |

# Makeup for the
## clear dominant

You have no problem wearing clear, bright colors in your 40s and can still do so if you are in your 50s or 60s and beyond. Older women just need to lighten up on the application.

## Combinations

### in your 40s

| Eye pencil | Lip pencil |
|---|---|
| soft black | red |

| Eye shadows | Lip colors |
|---|---|
| aqua | strawberry |
| cocoa | warm pink |
| steel | mango |
| Indian ocean | Blusher |
| | muscat |

### in your 50s

| Eye pencil | Lip pencil |
|---|---|
| petrol | cantaloupe |

| Eye shadows | Lip colors |
|---|---|
| melon | coral |
| mercury | fiesta |
| smoke | alfresco |
| peppermint | Blusher |
| | marsala |

### in your 60s and beyond

| Eye pencil | Lip pencil |
|---|---|
| granite | natural |

| Eye shadows | Lip colors |
|---|---|
| peach | breeze |
| pewter | spiced peach |
| delph | tulip |
| pearl | Blusher |
| | muscat |

# Makeup for the
## soft dominant

When applying your colors, do not forget to blend them really well. This is vital to maintaining harmony with your natural coloring, and particularly important when working on the eyes.

## Combinations

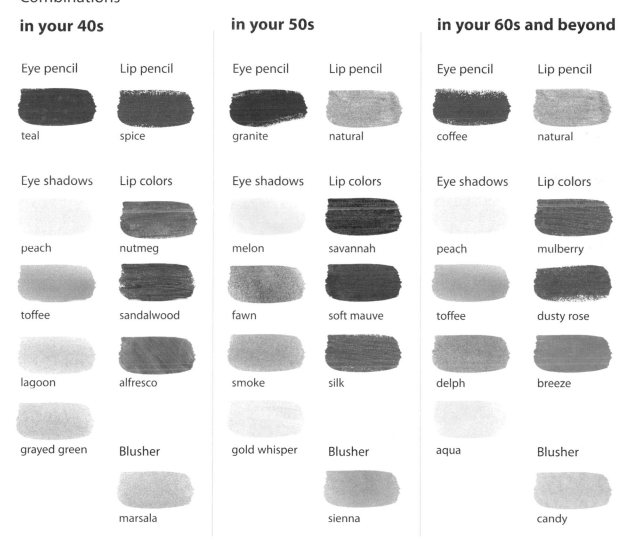

### in your 40s

| Eye pencil | Lip pencil |
| teal | spice |

| Eye shadows | Lip colors |
| peach | nutmeg |
| toffee | sandalwood |
| lagoon | alfresco |
| grayed green | **Blusher** |
| | marsala |

### in your 50s

| Eye pencil | Lip pencil |
| granite | natural |

| Eye shadows | Lip colors |
| melon | savannah |
| fawn | soft mauve |
| smoke | silk |
| gold whisper | **Blusher** |
| | sienna |

### in your 60s and beyond

| Eye pencil | Lip pencil |
| coffee | natural |

| Eye shadows | Lip colors |
| peach | mulberry |
| toffee | dusty rose |
| delph | breeze |
| aqua | **Blusher** |
| | candy |

# Good hair days

Your hair is your crowning glory, and you should make the most of it. A host of hair challenges hit you in your 40s, 50s, 60s, and beyond, and this gives you an opportunity to look at yourself afresh and reinvent yourself regularly.

Like skin, hair is affected by the hormonal changes that take place as you get older. It can change in texture, its color will change, and it may even thin out. Nothing dates you more than an outdated hairstyle. The good thing about hair is that it grows. If you don't like a cut or treatment, it is never too long before you can have another style or color.

You already know about bad hair days and how they can affect the way you feel all day. In order to move toward good hair days, you must learn about your face shape, what hairstyle suits you, the type of hair you have, and how you can look after it on a daily basis. On the following pages are guidelines on finding out your face shape and what hairstyles might suit you and your hair type in order to stay looking younger.

### Choosing a hairdresser

This may require some research. Ask a friend with a good haircut for a recommendation or stand outside a hair salon and see how women behave and look as they come out (are they smiling and feeling tall, or are they head down and fiddling with their hair?). A good hairdresser will always give you a short consultation before you book your first appointment and thereafter every time before shampooing. Don't feel anxious about telling your hairdresser if you don't like the end result.

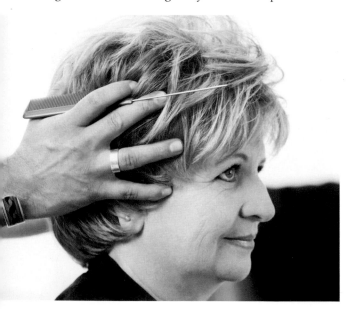

**If your ears tend to stick out a little, a close-cropped hairstyle will make them appear larger, so go for volume around the ears. If you have a large nose, add volume to the back of your hair to balance the look.**

Choose your hairdresser very carefully—he or she will make or break your look.

# What shape is your face?

The most balanced face shape is oval, and this is the shape that can wear any hairstyle. When hairdressers look at you, therefore, they will endeavor to create the illusion of an oval with the combination of your hair and face.

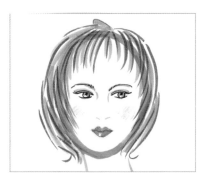

### An **oval** face
- Your face is wider at the cheekbones.
- It gently narrows down to a soft, rounded jawline and chin.

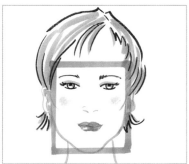

### A **square** face
- You have a wide forehead.
- Your face is straight from the cheekbones to the jawline and straight across the chin.
- It is even in width and length.

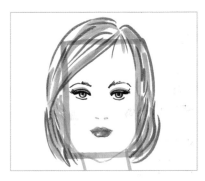

### A **rectangular** face
- Your face is straight from the cheekbones to the jawline and straight across the chin.
- It is longer than it is wide.

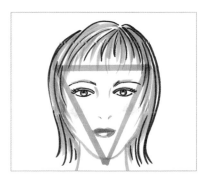

### An **inverted triangle** face
- You have a broad forehead and cheekbones.
- Your face tapers sharply to a pointed chin.

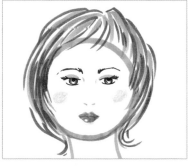

### A **round** face
- You have a narrow forehead.
- You have fuller cheekbones.
- You have a soft jawline and a soft chin.

### Necks, ears, and noses

The length and width of your neck will have a bearing on how long you can wear your hair. If you have a short, wide neck, keep the area clear. Check out what your hairstyle does to your profile to make sure it balances your head.

# Basic hairstyles

All hairstyles are taken from four basic haircuts and will often be a combination of elements from more than one of them. Although fashion may change and styles vary, these basic haircuts remain the same.

Once you have a hairstyle that suits you, ask your hairdresser to show you different ways of styling it, finishing it, and achieving the look yourself.

The sign of a good haircut is that it can be left without any styling and will still have a natural, relaxed, and young appearance. You will therefore still look presentable, even if for some reason you are unable to dry or style your own hair.

## Keeping your hair long

If you wear your hair long, make sure you keep it in excellent condition and trim it regularly. Extremely long hair is not a youthful look. If you wear it up, make sure you use good-quality pins, bands, and combs. How you wear your hair up will depend on your face shape, head shape, and lifestyle.

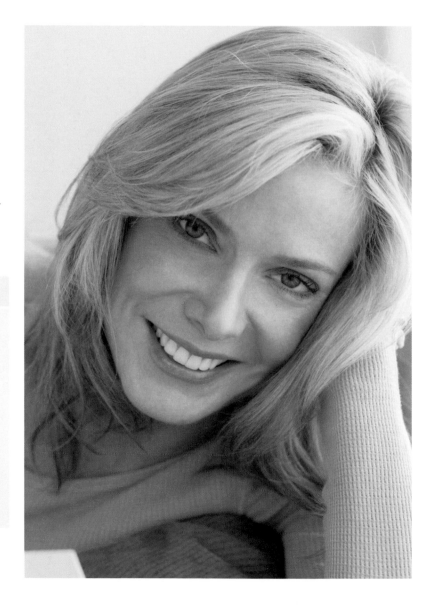

Choose a hairstyle that you can easily manage yourself on a daily basis.

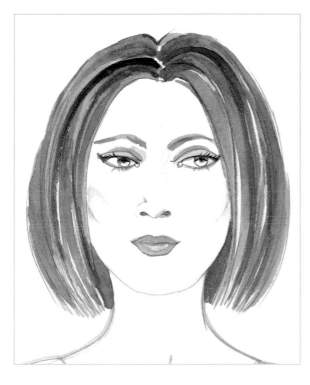

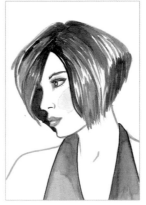

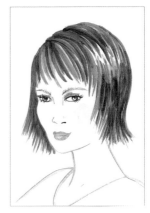

## One-length bob

In this cut, all the hair is the same length.

**Variations:**

• A graduated bob, which is shorter at the nape and longer at the jaw.

• A layered bob, where the bottom edge is one length, with long layers through it.

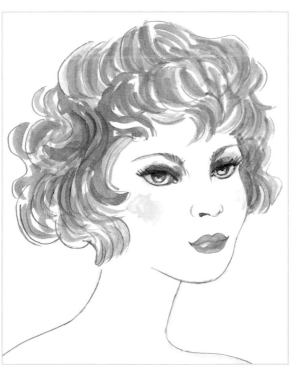

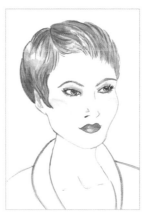

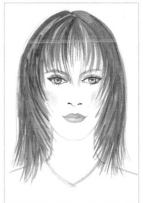

## Uniform layer

The hair is cut into short, even-length layers, which follow the shape of the head.

**Variations:**

• The pixie, which is short-cropped tight and to the head.

• Longer layers shaped evenly around the head.

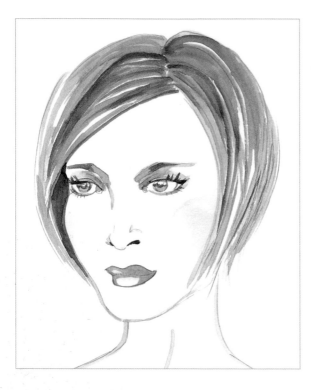

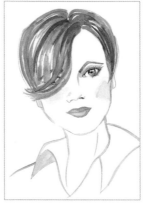

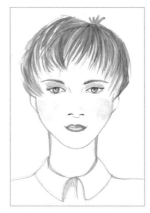

## Short graduation

The fullest part of the hair is at the temple and is then shaped into the nape area.

**Variations:**

• The wedge, which is a longer, softer version.

• The layered wedge, where the weight is at the temple, is layered at the crown and shaped into the nape.

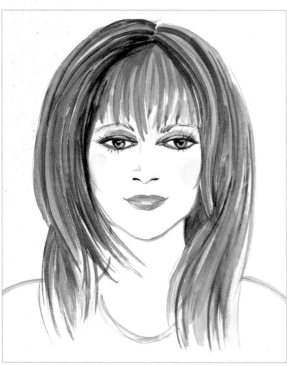

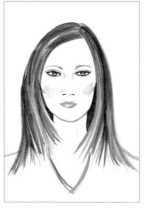

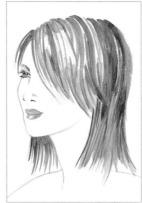

## Long layers

This is a style for long hair, with the shortest layer finishing at the nape.

**Variations:**

• Long, smooth graduations that are shaped at the front edge.

• Square layers, where the overall shape appears to be uneven.

# Making an **oval face** look younger

By the time you reach your 40s, your face may have become slightly more angular around the jawline and you will have lost some of the fullness from your cheeks, too. These changes will also be evident in your 50s, 60s, and beyond.

## Tips

✓ Allow your cheekbones to be seen with all styles.

✓ If you need more volume, use mousse before you dry your hair.

✓ If you need less volume, use a finishing product.

✗ Avoid heavy bangs.

✗ Avoid too much hair coming onto the face.

All you need to do is enhance the perfect shape of your face. The choice of hairstyle comes down to whether your hair is straight or curly.

## Hairstyles
• The one-length bob for straight hair.
• The uniform layer for curly hair.
• The short graduation for straight hair.
• Long layers for curly hair.

## Long hair
Have fun putting your hair up, and try using accessories to take it from a daytime to an evening look.

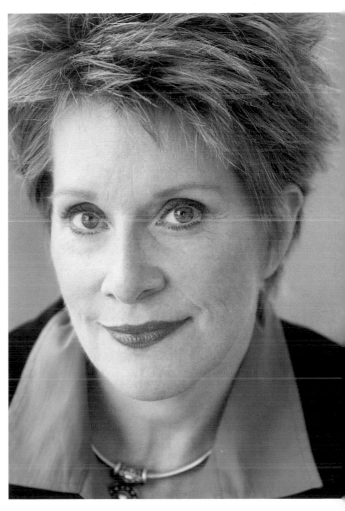

By keeping your hairstyle up to date and manageable, you can look both healthy and youthful.

# Making a **square face** look younger

You are likely to find that aging has made your jaw appear heavier than it did in previous decades. This is because you tend to lose tissue here in your 40s and beyond.

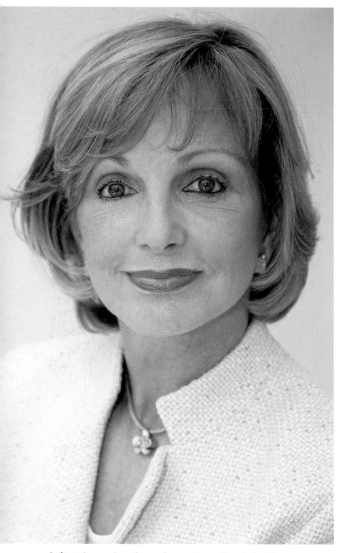

Soften the angles of your face with a softer hairstyle.

## Tips

✓ Use a finishing product such as wax to define the layers and soften the overall look.

✓ If you have a deep forehead, feathered or asymmetric bangs will be youthful.

✗ Avoid a one-length bob that finishes at the jawline.

✗ Avoid full, heavy, straight bangs.

You need to add width to the cheekbones and soften the angles of your forehead. You can achieve this by choosing a hairstyle that finishes at the cheekbones, possibly with a side part and a little length at the back of the neck.

## Hairstyles
• The uniform layer will give a rounded shape.
• The short graduation will add length at the nape.
• Long layers, with feathering onto the face, will soften the edge of your face.

## Long hair
Wear your hair up with fullness around the hairline and allow for some softness at the temples. The bulk of the hair should sit on the crown. If wearing it down, have fullness at the temples.

# Making a **rectangular face** look younger

You will find that the fullness of your cheeks has diminished a little over the years, and that you now have a slightly hollowed-out appearance that gives your face an even longer look.

## Tips

✓ Keep your hair shoulder length.

✓ Use a mousse at the roots before drying.

✓ Try to dry your hair with your head down to get root lift at the side.

✗ Don't wear long hair tight to the face (like a curtain).

✗ Avoid a middle part.

You need to add width to the side of your face and shorten its appearance by wearing hair on the forehead. This can be achieved by any kind of bangs or sweeping hair across to the side if wearing a part.

## Hairstyles
• The layered bob, flicked out, will give width to your face.
• The uniform layer will soften and give your face more width.
• Long layers to shoulder length will soften your face shape.
• The short graduation will accentuate the cheekbones, adding width to your face.
• The wedge will add fullness to your cheekbones, giving the illusion of shortening your face.

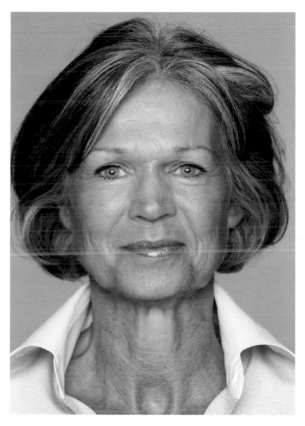

A rectangular face will benefit from a hairstyle with volume at the side and not on the top.

## Long hair
Allow for softness at the hairline by not pulling your hair back tightly. Wear the bulk of your hair at the nape or on the back of the head, not on top of the head.

# Making an **inverted triangle face** look younger

You will find that your face shape has not changed much with age. Nevertheless, you still need to reduce the width of your forehead and add fullness to the jawline to achieve a younger look.

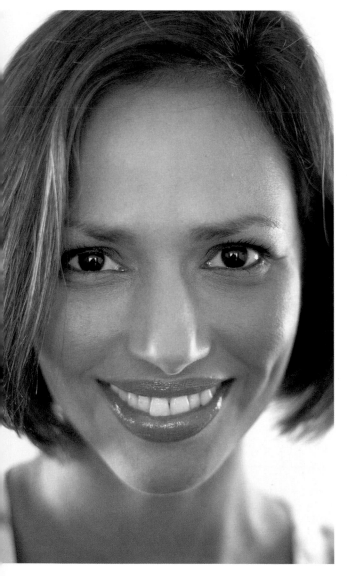

## Tips

✓ Try wispy bangs as an alternative to heavy, one-length bangs.

✓ Build up the texture and volume of the ends of the hair at chin level by using a finishing cream or hairspray.

✗ Avoid a very full hairstyle at the temples.

✗ Don't choose to have very short hairstyles.

## Hairstyles
• The graduated bob with bangs will narrow the width of your forehead.
• The layered bob with soft curls or flicked out will add width to your jawline.
• Long layers will balance your wide forehead.

## Long hair
You are better off keeping your hair down in long layers that can be flicked out at chin level to balance your wider forehead. If wearing your hair up, keep some hair to the sides of your forehead, but pull the rest back tight to the nape or back of your head.

If wearing a bob style, make sure it finishes at the jawline to add width to your face.

# Making a **round face** look younger

Whether you are in your 40s, 50s, or 60s and beyond, you will find that you have kept your youthful look longer than any woman of the same age who has a face of a different shape.

## Tips

✓ Keep your hair under control and the volume down with serums, waxes, and hairsprays.

✓ Try tucking your hair behind your ears.

✗ Don't have a center part.

✗ Avoid full bangs.

You need to counteract the roundness of your face by having hairstyles with straight lines and angles. Play down the volume if your hair is curly.

## Hairstyles
• The one-length bob will straighten the edges of your face.
• The graduated bob will give an angled appearance to your profile.
• A short graduation will accentuate your cheekbones, reducing roundness.
• A pixie haircut, for straight hair only.
• Long layers, if the crown area is kept sleek.

## Long hair
When putting your hair up, sweep it from one side to the other and gather it at the nape to give an asymmetrical look. If you have straight hair, gather it together and spike it up for a modern look.

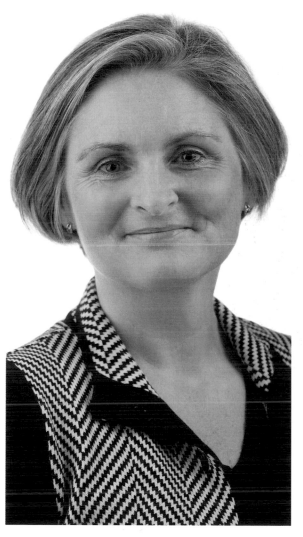

A straight style is a great way to wear your hair when you have a round face, because it complements its fullness.

# Having healthy hair

Without a doubt, your crowning glory needs care. Choosing the right products to use might seem overwhelming, but a little know-how can help your hair stay healthy for longer.

## When to use products

External elements—extreme weather conditions, swimming in the ocean or in a pool—will have an immediate effect on your hair, making it dry and brittle, that can easily be remedied with conditioners and serums. Medical treatments and stress may take longer to have an effect on your hair, but need to be addressed nonetheless. Regular use of product(s) tends to build up on the hair shaft, so vary the products from time to time to ensure that your hair stays healthy and shiny.

## What products to use

Separate shampoos and conditioners are best for your hair, as combined products build up quicker. Use products for your type of hair—for example, dry, normal, oily, or colored.

### Styling products

You can buy a host of additional products for styling your hair. Always apply them when the hair is wet.
• Mousse adds volume.
• Blow-dry lotions protect hair from the heat of dryers and rollers.
• Setting lotion holds your hairstyle in place.
• Serums control dryness and frizz.

### Finishing products

These are best used on dry hair.
• Wax gives definition to your hair ends.
• Dressing creams keep your style in place and add shine.
• Shine spray adds gloss to your hair.
• Hairspray holds your hair in place.

## Getting curly

To add body and volume to your hair, you may want to have a perm. Nowadays these will give you added volume and a gentle wave to the hair to allow movement. Fashion often dictates whether to choose a tight curl or a loose wave. If you keep your hair permed, you'll need regular treatment,

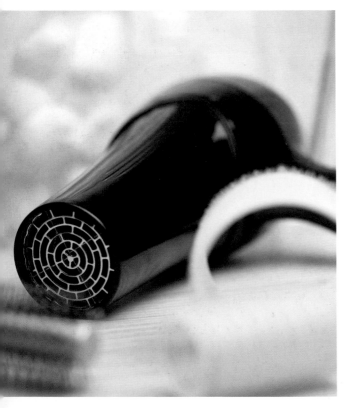

Good tools will allow you to style your hair with a salon-finished flair.

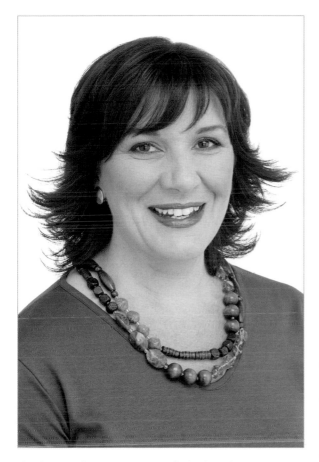

The three Cs of hair care are cut, color, and condition.

## Tips for your hair type

### Fine
- Use a volumizing shampoo.
- Use mousse to add and maintain volume.
- Avoid wax-based products.

### Thick
- Use a conditioner to smooth your hair.
- Use wax to separate hairs and define your hairstyle.
- Choose a haircut that reduces the volume.

### Curly
- Use a moisturizing shampoo and conditioner.
- Use a serum to control frizz.
- If using a straightening iron, use a lotion to protect your hair from the heat.

### Thinning
- Use a volumizing shampoo.
- Have a regular head massage to stimulate the roots, which encourages hair growth.
- Keep your hairstyle relatively short.

### Colored
- Use shampoos and conditioners for colored hair.
- Use a styling product to give sheen.
- Keep up the color.

depending on how fast your hair grows. You can also use tongs and heated rollers for instant curls.

For an instant change to your look try some large foam rollers, which are wound into your hair. After you remove the rollers, brush your hair thoroughly for a glamorous look.

## Getting straight

Over the past few years, chemical straightening has become more and more popular and successful, but it does need to be done by a professional. You can use straightening irons for a temporary solution, or to sleek down flyaway hair, but don't forget to use a serum or blow-drying product on your hair first.

## Hair dryers

It is worth investing in a professional hair dryer with a large narrow nozzle and a diffuser that allows you to style your hair. It should have a number of heat and speed settings. Test the weight of the hair dryer to make sure you can hold it above your head for a period of time.

Giving your hair a cold blast at the end of drying will help your style last longer.

# Color for younger-looking hair

Your hair color is the key to a younger-looking you. Over the decades your hair will have lightened considerably. Basically, hair loses the ability to hold color and the shaft turns white. The more white hairs you have, the lighter your hair appears in general.

There are many different ways of adding color to your hair. The choice is how long you want it to last and whether you want to do it yourself or have it done by your hairdresser. Here are your options:
• Temporary color is available as a color mousse, setting lotion, or hairspray.
• Color-enhancing shampoo extends the life of an artificial color.
• Semipermanent color lasts for six to eight shampoos.
• Quasi, or demipermanent, color lasts for 12 to 24 shampoos.
• Permanent color covers white hair and needs to be colored as it regrows—every six weeks.

## Going gray

In hairdressing terms, there is no such thing as gray hair. "Gray" is simply the term used for hair that has a mixture of white hairs and hairs of the natural color. The hair looks gray because the natural color is seen through the white hair.

## Highlights and lowlights

These techniques involve coloring strands of hair using a permanent color. As the terms suggests, highlighting is when sections of hair are made lighter, while lowlighting is when the sections of hair are colored darker or the tone is changed. You can combine highlights and lowlights for a younger look. By changing the size of the sections colored, you can also add texture and volume to your hair.

## Block coloring

In block coloring, whole sections of hair are colored lighter or darker to define a cut. This is a great way to cover gray hair that might appear in just one area. It does need to be done by a professional, however.

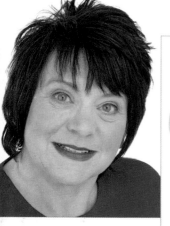
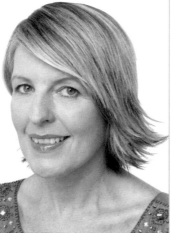

Lowlights (left) and highlights (right) will add texture and volume to your hair. They will also make any artificial coloring appear more natural.

# Hair color basics

When your hair starts to change color, there are several options open to you (see below). In all cases, you need to consider both depth and undertone and how your new color will affect your dominant.

Women in their 40s, 50s, 60s, and beyond often allow their hair to go white, naturally and gracefully, and change their dominant accordingly. If this is not for you, consider one of the following routes: color your white hair with a tint to match your natural color (keeping your dominant the same); or color the 'gray'—that is all your hair—a different color (thereby changing your dominant).

If you like your gray hair you might want to add cool tones to enhance the color. Your budget and your own skills will determine whether you go to a hairdresser to achieve the color that you want, or whether you do it yourself at home. The hair color samples shown here will vary, depending on your natural color and how much gray there is.

## Depth

The chart below shows the depth of color from 10 (the lightest) to 1 (the darkest). If you want to change the color of your hair, and want the new color to be natural looking, you should go no more than two shades above or below your own hair color. If you are completely white, do not go darker than your natural coloring: go back to your natural depth or lighter.

## Undertone

If your hair had natural warm tones that have faded, consider reintroducing warm tones to your hair.

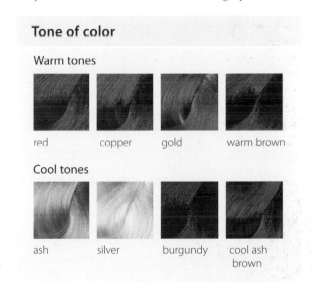

### Tone of color

**Warm tones**

| red | copper | gold | warm brown |

**Cool tones**

| ash | silver | burgundy | cool ash brown |

## Depth of color

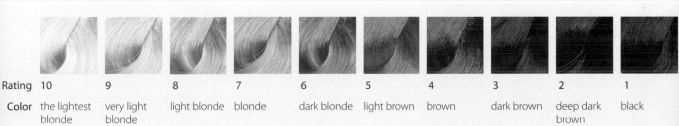

| Rating | 10 | 9 | 8 | 7 | 6 | 5 | 4 | 3 | 2 | 1 |
|--------|----|----|----|----|----|----|----|----|----|----|
| Color | the lightest blonde | very light blonde | light blonde | blonde | dark blonde | light brown | brown | dark brown | deep dark brown | black |

# Hair color options for the
## light dominant

You are a natural blonde, and over the years you may have added a little color. Your hair tends to be fine, so adding highlights will not only enhance the color but will add texture to your hair, too.

## Depth

One shade up or down will be adequate (see page 99). It is advisable to go darker, because your skin and eye color remain light.

## Tone

You can enhance the tone of your hair by adding a cool or warm tone, depending on your skin color.

### The best colors for you

  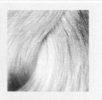

**In your 40s**
Very light natural golden blonde

**In your 50s**
Lightest blonde

**In your 60s and beyond**
Lightest pale ash blonde

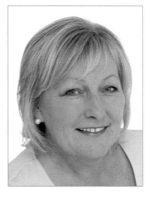 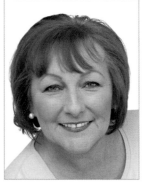

Here the hair has been warmed with gold tones, changing the dominant from light to warm.

### Changing your dominant

| Natural hair color | Blonde | Ash blonde |
|---|---|---|
| Eye color | Blue or green | Blue-gray |
| Skin color | Freckled and delicate | Rosy and delicate |
| New hair color (natural or with tint) | Add copper or gold tones | White, silver, or ash |
| New dominant | Warm | Cool |

# Hair color options for the
## deep dominant

With your dark coloring, you have the choice of adding warm or cool lowlights. The amount of gray in your hair will determine how long you can go on tinting you hair.

### Depth
Your dark eyes will prevent you from going more than two shades lighter (see page 99).

### Tone
For warm tones, you could add red or copper; for cool tones, you could add cool brown or burgundy.

**The best colors for you**

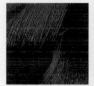  

In your 40s
Dark brown

In your 50s
Medium brown

In your 60s and beyond
Light brown

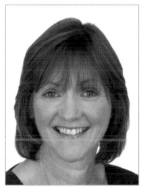 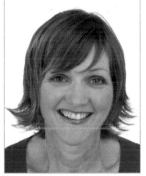

The natural highlights have been covered with a dark blonde tint, making our deep model soft.

**Changing your dominant**

| | | | |
|---|---|---|---|
| Natural hair color | Dark brown | Dark brown | Dark brown |
| Eye color | Dark brown or black | Dark brown or black | Dark brown or black |
| Skin color | Porcelain to black | Porcelain to black | Porcelain to black |
| New hair color (natural or with tint) | Add copper and red tones to give you auburn hair | You keep your hair white | Add a dark blonde tint to go dark blonde or light brown |
| New dominant | Warm | Cool | Soft |

# Hair color options for the
# warm dominant

Whether you are strawberry blonde or dark auburn, your hair will always benefit from having warm tones added to it to maintain the harmony with your natural skin and eye coloring.

## Depth
You have the choice of going lighter or of keeping the same color, depending on how much gray there is (see page 99).

## Tone
Use gold, copper, or red to enhance your natural hair color.

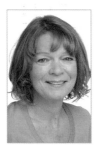 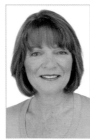

For a youthful soft dominant use a dark blonde tint to cover the gray.

### The best colors for you

| In your 40s | In your 50s | In your 60s and beyond |
|---|---|---|
| Medium golden blonde | Light golden blonde | Lightest golden blonde |

| Deep copper | Golden copper | Light copper |

## Changing your dominant

| | | | |
|---|---|---|---|
| Natural hair color | Strawberry blonde | Auburn | Auburn |
| Eye color | Blue, green, or amber | Blue, green, amber, or brown | Blue, green, amber, or brown |
| Skin color | Freckled or golden | Freckled or golden | Freckled or golden |
| New hair color (natural or with tint) | Naturally light blonde | Naturally pure white | Use a dark blonde tint to cover the gray, or keep to a salt-and-pepper look |
| New dominant | Light | Cool | Soft |

# Hair color options for the
## cool dominant

Women with cool coloring can be anything from white- to dark-haired. The key for you is to keep any tint cool and to resist the temptation to add any warm tone.

## Depth
You should stay within the two shades rule (see page 99), but can go either lighter or darker.

## Tone
Cool brown, ash, silver, and light burgundy are all colors that work well for you.

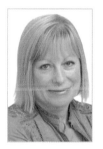
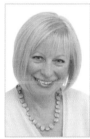

Add an ash blonde tint to achieve a light dominant, which is more youthful.

### The best colors for you

| In your 40s | In your 50s | In your 60s and beyond |
|---|---|---|
| Dark ash brown | Medium ash brown | Light ash brown |

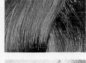

| Light ash blonde | Very light ash blonde | Lightest ash blonde |
|---|---|---|

### Changing your dominant

| Natural hair color | Ash blonde | Ash brown/black |
|---|---|---|
| Eye color | Blue-gray | Blue, gray, or brown |
| Skin color | Cool undertones (rosy) | Cool undertones (rosy) |
| New hair color (natural or with tint) | Naturally light ash blonde | Add an ash tint to cover the gray, making you a light ash brown or dark blonde |
| New dominant | Light | Soft |

# Hair color options for the
# clear dominant

To keep your clear look, and therefore stay looking younger, your hair needs to be kept dark. You need to consider whether a change in your dominant is more age-appropriate.

## Depth

If your hair is brown and you go lighter, you will change your dominant coloring (see below).

## Tone

You have the choice of either going warm (red, copper, warm brown) or cool (ash brown or burgundy).

### The best colors for you

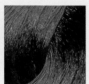

**In your 40s**
Dark brown

**In your 50s**
Medium brown

**In your 60s and beyond**
Light brown

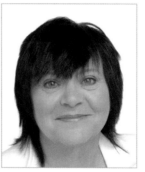
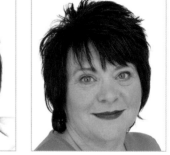

Adding lowlights to an overall color will give you a more youthful look.

### Changing your dominant

| Natural hair color | Dark | Dark | Dark | Dark |
|---|---|---|---|---|
| Eye color | Green, blue, or topaz | Green, blue, or topaz | Green, blue, or topaz | Green, blue, or topaz |
| Skin color | Porcelain | Porcelain to black | Porcelain | Porcelain to black |
| New hair color (natural or with tint) | You have plenty of gray and are now tinting it light blonde | You already have some red in your hair, and you've added a warm tint to it, making you auburn | Naturally pure white | You have covered the gray to become light brown or dark blonde |
| New dominant | Light | Warm | Cool | Soft |

# Hair color options for the
## soft dominant

Your hair color has changed from dark blonde to light brown, and will now benefit from having highlights added in order for you to maintain a more youthful appearance.

## Depth
Your hair is medium depth, neither light nor dark.

## Tone
You can add warm (copper, gold) or cool shades (ash, silver), depending on your skin tone.

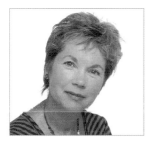 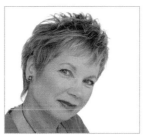

Adding warm gold tints has changed our model's dominant from soft to warm.

### The best colors for you

| In your 40s | In your 50s | In your 60s and beyond |
|---|---|---|
| Dark blonde | Blonde | Light blonde |

| Light brown | Dark blonde | Blonde |
|---|---|---|

### Changing your dominant

| | | | |
|---|---|---|---|
| **Natural hair color** | Light brown or dark blonde | Light brown or dark blonde | Dark blonde |
| **Eye color** | Muted blue, green, or hazel | Muted blue, green or hazel | Muted blue, green, or hazel |
| **Skin color** | Neutral | Golden tones | Rosy |
| **New hair color** (natural or with tint) | You have plenty of gray and are now tinting it light blonde | You have covered the gray with copper or gold | You have covered the gray with ash tones or have gone naturally gray |
| **New dominant** | Light | Warm | Cool |

# A younger look with glasses

You may have escaped wearing glasses in your youth. However, by the time you reach your 40s and beyond, the lens of the eye begins to deteriorate (presbyopia) and regular eye exams are necessary to make sure you don't suffer from eyestrain.

The good news is that glasses have become something of a fashion accessory. Think about having several frames for different occasions—daytime, evening wear, sunshine. Of course, you also have the option of wearing contact lenses. If you only need reading glasses, these are available over the counter in all sorts of styles and colors.

When choosing a frame, you need to consider your face shape, your coloring, and your lifestyle. Go for a frame that will work with these as well as with your prescription. Glasses are an investment buy, so make sure you get them right.

## Choosing your frames

**A good fit:** Your optician should make sure your glasses fit you properly. If they start to slide down your nose, go back and have them tightened again.
**The bridge:** This is the area of the glasses that rests on your nose. Note the placement of the bridge when you try on a frame. On a long nose, the bridge should be low down, while on a short nose, the bridge should be higher.
**Scale and proportion:** You need to consider the dimensions of a frame, and this will depend on your face shape and size. Larger facial features demand a heavier-looking frame, while small and delicate features demand a lighter-looking one.

## Lenses

Varifocals are lenses that are graduated for different prescriptions, to allow you to see distance and

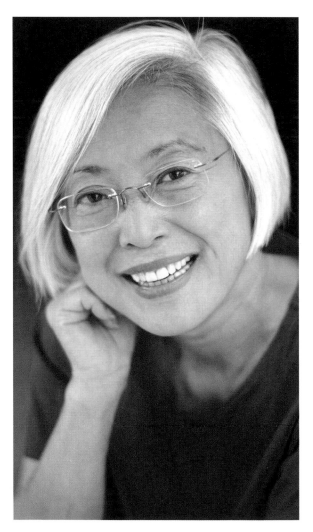

Balance the style of your frames with your coloring, face shape, and scale.

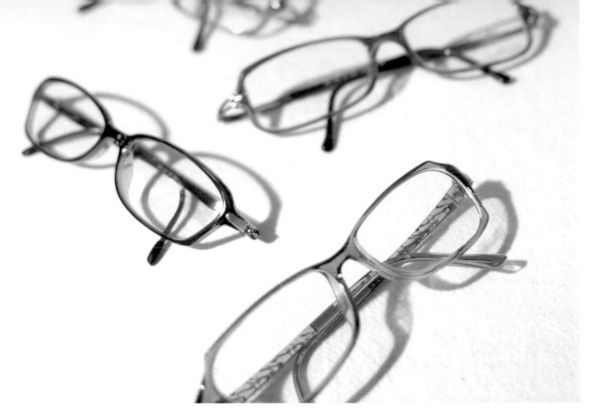

Choose frames in a color that works with your wardrobe.

close up. This is a much better alternative to bifocal lenses (showing a visible line), which are aging.

Transition lenses (or reactions) are an excellent alternative to having two pairs of glasses—one for the sun and one for inside. These lenses are photochromic and react to the light, darkening to offer protection when exposed to bright light.

You can buy prescription sunglasses, although these are often regarded as a fashion item.

## Glasses and makeup

Depending on your prescription, the lenses of your glasses will vary, and this will affect how others see your eye through the lens. Here are some easy and simple makeup tips to minimize any distortions caused by the lenses.

### You are nearsighted

This means the lenses in your glasses will make your eyes appear smaller. To remedy this, you should use a light or bright eye pencil color around

### Tip

If you are farsighted and have difficulty seeing things close up, applying makeup can become challenging. You need good light and a magnifying mirror to see what you are doing.

the eye and keep the eye shadow colors light. Avoid dark and black eyeliner, which will make your eyes look even smaller, but do double-layer your mascara.

### You are farsighted

This means the lenses in your glasses will make your eyes appear larger. To remedy this, you should use the darker or more muted shades from your palette. Avoid bright or strong colors, as these will make the eye appear even larger. Use concealer or skin adjuster under the eye, since dark circles will also be magnified.

## Contact lenses

Contact lenses are great for removing the barrier that is often created when wearing glasses, and for encouraging good eye contact. Your eyes will also appear slightly more sparkling and healthier, giving a younger look. If you are tempted to use contact lenses to change the natural color of your eyes, be aware that this might also change your dominant coloring characteristic.

## The right color glasses

If you wear glasses, the color of your frames needs to balance with your dominant coloring type. Choose them well, and your glasses will harmonize with your entire wardrobe.

Using your color palette as a guide, select neutral colors if you intend to have just one pair of glasses. If you are selecting a fashion pair, choose one of your fashion colors. You could also consider rimless or semirimless glasses, which are now an

excellent alternative, especially if they are fitted with nonreflective lenses. These frames can be worn for any occasion and with any color. Embellishments on frames are fun but can quickly date them, so it may not be a wise investment.

## Getting the shape right

Your face shape will dictate the best shape of glasses for you (see page 87). Take time when making a choice. If necessary, go to more than one optician until you find what works best for you.

### An oval face

Yours is the most balanced face, so most frame styles will suit you. Make sure that the scale of the frames balances with the scale of your face, and avoid frames with extreme angles.

### A square face

You need to give width to your face by extending the width of the frames and softening the lines. Try oval or rounded shapes.

### A rectangular face

Wider frames with a low bridge will give the illusion of shortening the face. Avoid sharp angles on your frames. Wide arms will "break up" the length of the face, giving the illusion of shortening your face.

### An inverted triangle face

Keep the size of the frame within the width of your face. Rimless frames are good, as are semirimless frames where the rim is on the bottom half.

### A round face

Angled frames are good, as are those that are slightly wider than your face, but avoid heavy, rounded frames. A straight bridge is better than one that is curved.

Choosing the right shape of frames will give the appearance of a well-proportioned face.

### What color suits you?

| Dominant | Suitable colors |
| --- | --- |
| Light | pewter, taupe, cream, silver, gold, rimless |
| Deep | black, chocolate, olive, silver, gold, semirimless |
| Warm | chocolate, olive, amber, bronze, semirimless |
| Cool | charcoal, navy, purple, pewter, silver, rimless |
| Clear | black, scarlet, royal blue, silver, gold, semirimless |
| Soft | rose brown, charcoal blue, grayed green, silver, gold, rimless |

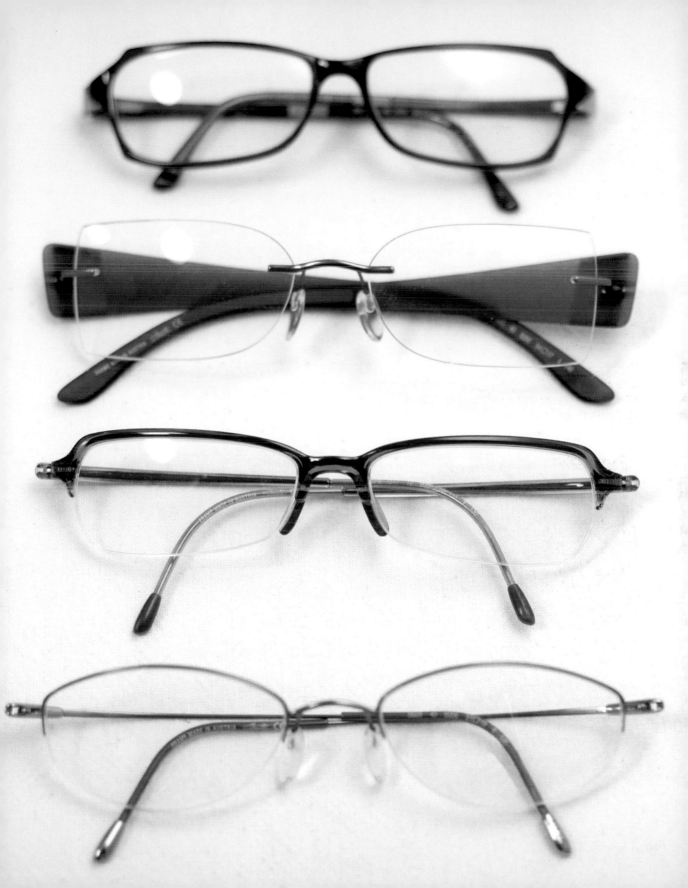

# A younger
# body

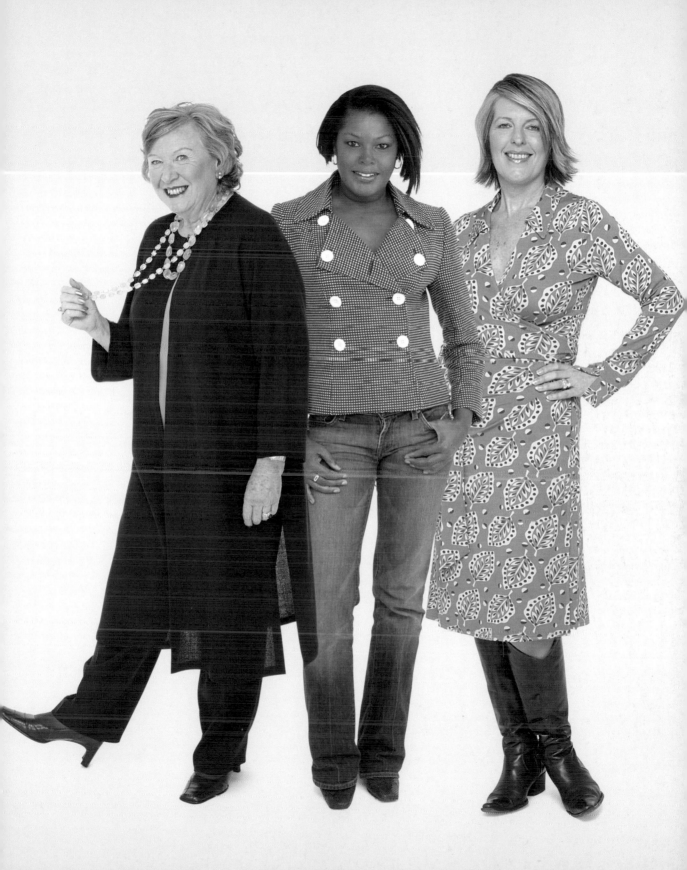

# Body maintenance

No matter what your age, your body—and that includes your hands and feet—needs a regular skincare routine of cleansing, exfoliating, and nourishing. If you do not already have a routine, now is the time to start one.

## Why body maintenance?

Often as we age the demands on our time lessen, so why not use this new free time on a little self-pampering? This can be done as a special treat at a spa or beauty salon or at home. We sometimes neglect our body, thinking that it is only our face that needs the attention. By having a well-cared-for body, not only will you feel better, but you will glow with self-confidence from top to bottom.

## Cleansing and exfoliating

When choosing a soap, make sure that it is one that contains nutritious oils (avocado, shea butter, or almond, for example). As your skin gets drier, make sure that your shower gel is one with moisturizing properties.

When showering or bathing, it is a good idea to exfoliate with a body brush, a loofah, or a

**Treat yourself to a body massage. They help the circulation, ease muscular aches and pains, and can generally have a beneficial effect on your well-being.**

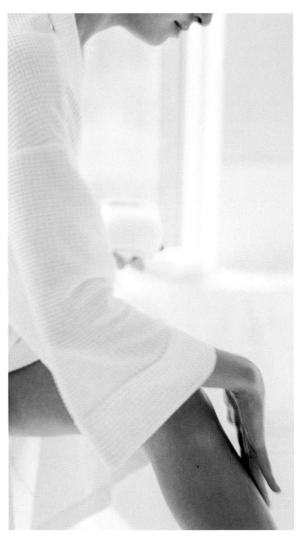

A little pampering can give you a great psychological lift and put a spring in your step.

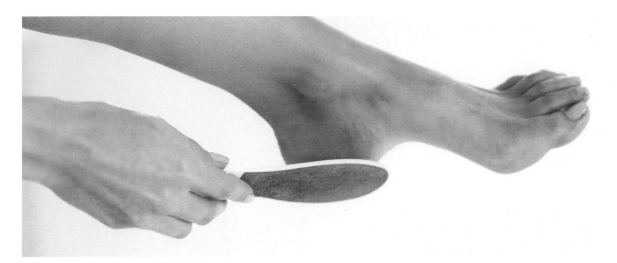

product to remove dead skin cells from your body, paying special attention to elbows, knees, and heels. Drying yourself briskly with a towel will also remove dead skin cells and improve circulation.

Apply body lotion to smooth and hydrate your skin. If you have particularly dry skin, use a cream. Pay special attention to your cleavage, as this tends to lose its elasticity first. Elbows and knees also need special attention.

If you have a favorite fragrance, think about layering by using shower cream/soap, body cream, deodorant, and talc as well as the fragrance itself.

## Body hair

Visible body hair is unattractive at any age! The good news is that, as you get older, this becomes sparser and softer. Whether you choose to shave, wax, or use a depilatory cream is up to you and will depend on the hair growth. Don't forget to moisturize afterward.

## Manicures

Nails and hands are as much an indication of age as your face, so whether you have a professional manicure or do it yourself, it is an important part of your overall grooming. Adapt your nail length and color to your lifestyle.

Your feet take the brunt of your lifestyle, so they need to be looked after —buff and moisturize them regularly.

## Pedicures

As you get older, regular inspections of your feet and toenails might not be as easy as they used to be! A professional pedicure will not only give you glamorous feet, but will ensure that any changes to your feet will be noticed (ingrown toenails, fungus, calluses).

## Sun care

If at any time you expose any part of your body to the sun, you must protect it against the damaging ultraviolet (UVA/UVB) rays. Damage is not just superficial with burning or tanning of the skin; the UVB rays actually penetrate to the lower level of the skin and break down the elastin and collagen fibers. It is the major cause of premature aging and skin disease. So, whether you are walking to work, gardening, or just relaxing outside, *always* use a high factor sunscreen or block and remember that when it comes to the sun, less is best.

There are many excellent products for achieving an artificial tan without damaging your skin. Although your skin may tan a little and slightly change color, this does not change your dominant coloring characteristics.

# Dressing for a changing shape

There is no need to panic! Many a woman's body shape will change in her 40s and beyond. Good body maintenance and a healthy diet are key to your keeping a great-looking body; it takes time, devotion, and a budget.

The well-dressed woman understands how to deal with her changing shape, and realizes that she can maintain a stylish and current look if she goes for fitness and quality. You need to learn that established dressing trends are more important than high fashion and, under no circumstances should you try to emulate your daughter or popular style icons.

Getting older does not mean you leave fashion trends behind.

Understanding your basic body shape will allow you to make informed choices when it comes to choosing clothing that will flatter you and even make you look trimmer and younger. It is essential for you to be realistic about your good points and to learn how to dress to accommodate the less good ones. Often, what you wear underneath will make or break an outfit, and here you will learn to treat your underwear with as much consideration as you do the rest of your wardrobe.

A well-planned wardrobe will guarantee that you always have the right piece at hand, whatever the occasion. Having reached your 40s, 50s, 60s, and beyond, your shopping trips are probably less spontaneous and generally better organized. Read on for guidelines on the types of clothes you should be wearing, not only to flatter your body, but also that are appropriate for your age and lifestyle. At the end of the chapter you can also find answers to the most frequently asked questions at **colour me beautiful**.

If you don't enjoy buying clothes, you will know that the whole shopping experience quickly becomes a task you would rather put off. Once you have identified what suits you, however, shopping becomes so much easier and more pleasurable. And do not worry about the expense of dressing to look younger—you don't need a large budget to become a well-dressed woman! A core wardrobe of good basic pieces in your best neutrals means that just by adding a few well-chosen accessories or tops you will have a wardrobe that works for you, not against you.

# Body shapes

There are six basic body shapes. Look at the descriptions below and see which one best describes you. Don't be alarmed if you find you have one body shape for your top half, and another for your lower half—it certainly isn't unusual.

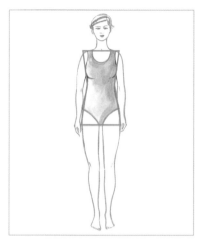

**Neat hourglass:** You wear the same top and bottom size, and have a waist.

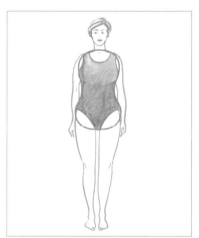

**Full hourglass:** Your bust is full, your hips are rounded; often waistbands on skirts and trousers are too big.

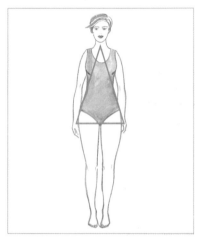

**Triangle:** You wear a smaller size on the top than on the bottom; you have full hips or thighs.

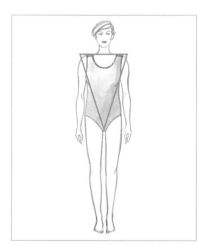

**Inverted triangle:** You wear a larger size on the top than on the bottom, and have narrow hips and a flat bottom.

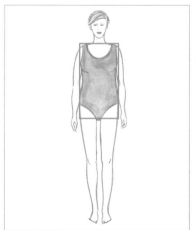

**Rectangle:** You have very little waist definition and a flat bottom and hips.

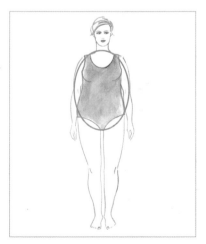

**Round:** You have rounded shoulder lines and a full waist and tummy.

# A younger neat hourglass body

You have the perfect body, and everyone envies you. Basically, you have the choice of most styles and shapes as long as your proportions are balanced. Even if you have crept up a size or two over the years, you still have a great body and should be proud to show it off whatever your age, as long as you wear an appropriate style. Avoid bulky fabrics and designs that hide your shape and don't show off your waist.

## Shape basics
- You have the perfect body shape.
- You have a defined waist.
- You find shopping easy.
- You have kept your youthful shape.

## What to wear

**Pants**  bootleg jeans • low-rise flares • palazzo • combats

**Skirts**  culottes • pencil • A-line • flipped • bias • narrow pleats

**Tops**  strapless • Bardot neckline • empire • fitted shirt • fitted sweater • wrap

**Dresses**  bias • belted • wrap • coat

**Jackets**  single-breasted • double-breasted • denim • shawl collar • safari

Wrap designs are easy to wear and are very flattering.

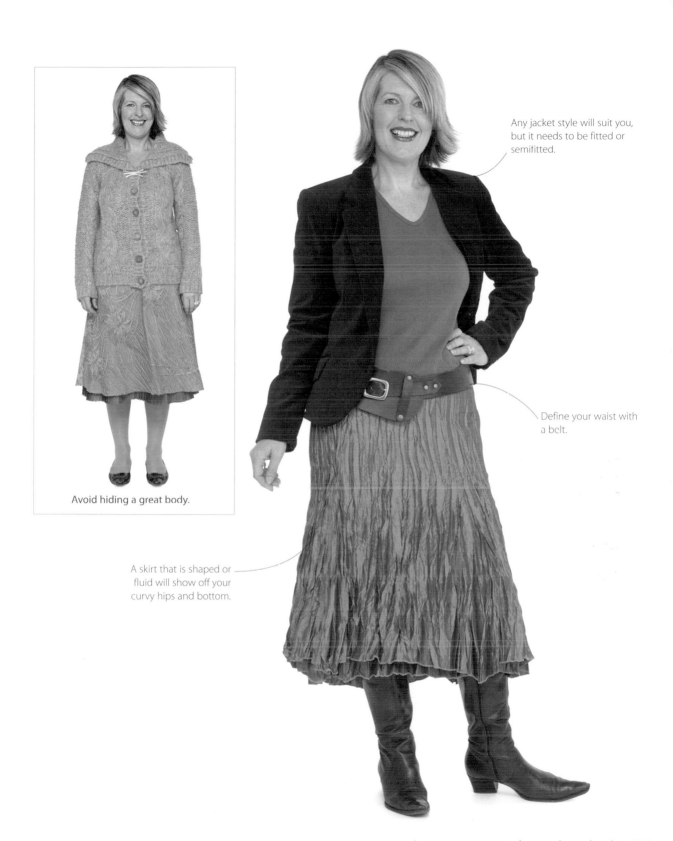

Avoid hiding a great body.

Any jacket style will suit you, but it needs to be fitted or semifitted.

Define your waist with a belt.

A skirt that is shaped or fluid will show off your curvy hips and bottom.

# A younger **full hourglass** body

You lucky voluptuous thing! You have a great choice of styles available to you. The most important thing for you to remember when shopping is to choose the right fabric. Whatever your size, your clothing line needs to follow the curves of your body with softer styling. Define the waist with belts or details, and make sure your clothes move with you.

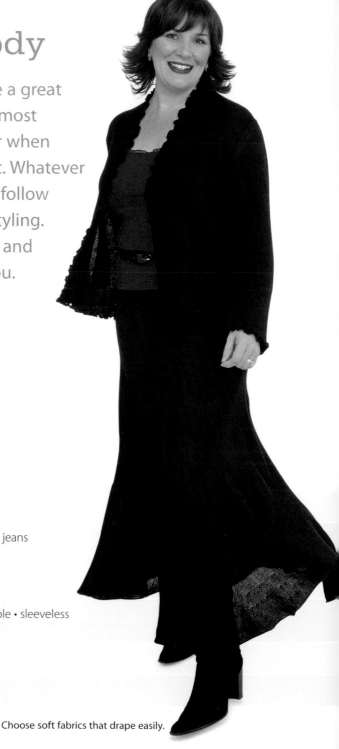

## Shape basics
- You have a very feminine figure.
- You have a full bust.
- You may have problems getting jackets and tops to fit over your bust.
- You may find that clothes that fit on the hips are too big on the waist.

## What to wear

**Pants**  flat-fronted • flared • palazzo • bootleg • drawstring • jeans (with no bottom details)

**Skirts**  flipped • bias • wrapped • tiered

**Tops**  scoop neck and V-neck wrap • fitted sweater • camisole • sleeveless turtleneck (long neck required) • gathered shirt

**Dresses**  bias • princess line • wrap • belted

**Jackets**  shawl collar • cardigan style

Choose soft fabrics that drape easily.

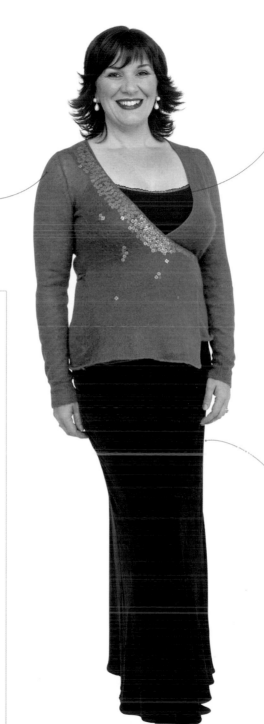

Knits are a wonderful addition to your wardrobe and make great alternatives to formal jackets.

Tank tops are great for ensuring that you don't expose too much cleavage.

Bias-cut skirts will fall smoothly over your wonderful full hips.

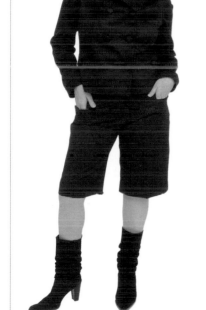

Avoid stiff, crisp fabrics and straight clothing lines.

# A younger
## triangle body

Whether you have a straight hip line or a curvy one, playing down this area is key. You are going to have fun adding details above the waistline, learning to layer and accessorize the top half of your body to give you the appearance of being in balance. Bright-colored details and texture draw the eye to the top half of your body. Pocket details and low-slung belts all draw attention to your hips and should be avoided at all costs.

## Shape basics
• You need to balance your body.
• You have wide hips.
• You have narrow shoulders.
• You may experience difficulty when buying dresses.

## What to wear

**Pants**  plain-fronted • bootleg • flared • palazzo

**Skirts**  pencil • flipped • bias • paneled

**Tops**  ruffle • twinset (for layering) • bulky sweater • shirts (with a camisole under) • waistcoat (with shirt and camisole under)

**Dresses**  wrap • empire • matching separates

**Jackets**  open-front • double-breasted • military • safari

Build up the top half of your body.

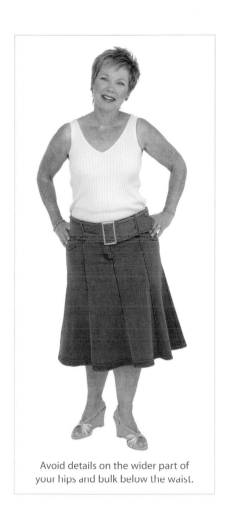

Avoid details on the wider part of your hips and bulk below the waist.

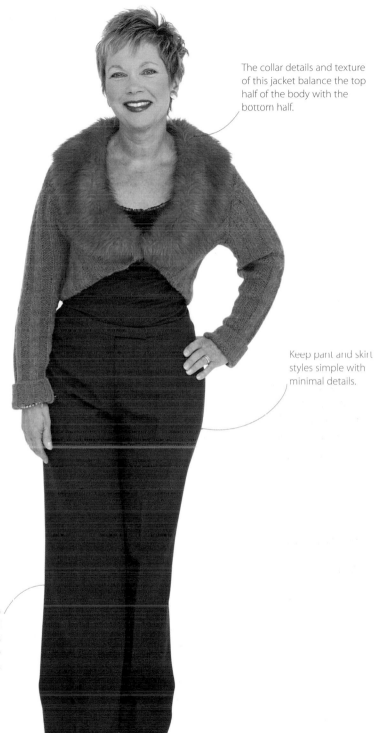

The collar details and texture of this jacket balance the top half of the body with the bottom half.

Keep pant and skirt styles simple with minimal details.

Add color to the top half of your body and wear darker neutrals below the waist to balance your figure.

# A younger **inverted triangle** body

Simple, uncluttered lines are your bywords.
Your clothing lines need to be straight and
angled. Crisper fabrics and tighter weaves
are just great on you. Adding details below
the waist will give you a more balanced look.
You will always look great in jeans and slacks.
Constructed lines and angled details enhance
your body shape. Soft, fluid fabrics and gathers
add bulk to your straight body lines and should
be avoided.

## Shape basics
• Your narrow hips are a great feature.
• You have straight, square shoulders.
• Your hips are trim and flat.
• You look good in pants.

## What to wear

**Pants** classic • jeans • cropped • bootleg • narrow

**Skirts** pencil • box pleats • paneled • denim-style • stitched-down pleats

**Tops** square and V-neck • halter neck • vest • fitted shirt • vest

**Dresses** shift • coat • low waist

**Jackets** open-front • double-breasted • denim

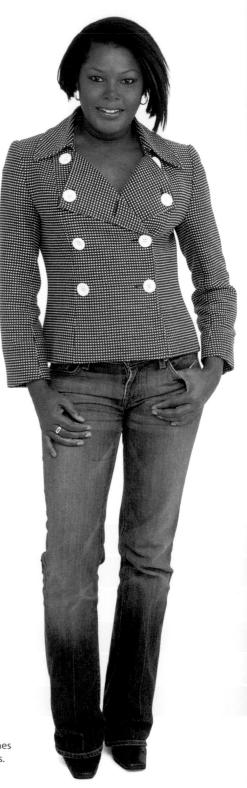

Stick to straight lines
with crisper fabrics.

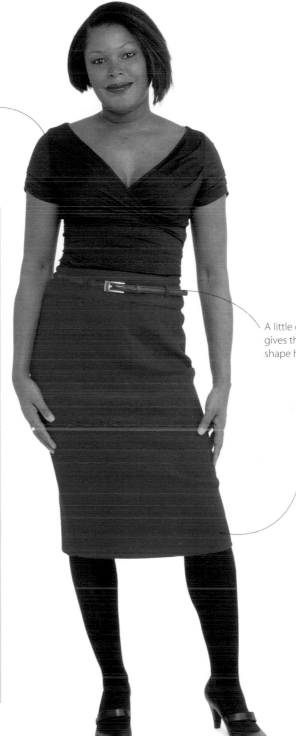

The lines of the neckline are straight and the top fitted, which enhances the shoulders and body line.

A little detail at the waist gives the illusion of some shape here.

A straight, fitted skirt shows off your slim figure.

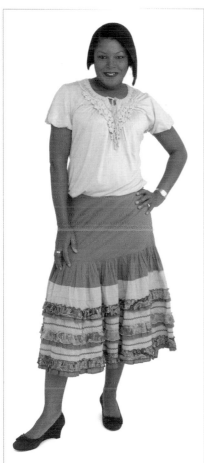

Avoid bulky, floppy clothing and florals or frills.

# A younger
# rectangle body

Your challenge is to give your body some curves, and you are in luck. It is easy to achieve the illusion of curves with the right clothes. But be aware that you can add years to your appearance if you get it wrong. Straight-line clothes with some shaping toward the waist will give you the figure you have always longed for. Don't be afraid of showing off your hips and bottom: they are your greatest assets.

## Shape basics
• You need to introduce some curves.
• You feel that you have no waist.
• You tend to carry extra weight around the middle.
• You have a flat bottom and hips

## What to wear

**Pants** front crease (to give a straight line) • flat-fronted • low-waisted • bootleg • jeans

**Skirts** pencil • paneled • box pleats • dropped panel

**Tops** square and V-necklines • semifitted shirt • shaped twinset • tank top

**Dresses** shift • coat • princess line • empire

**Jackets** single-breasted with lapels • double-breasted • open-front

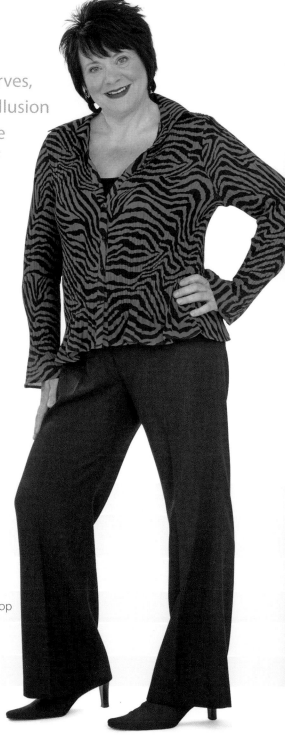

Clothing lines must remain straight, even in softer fabrics.

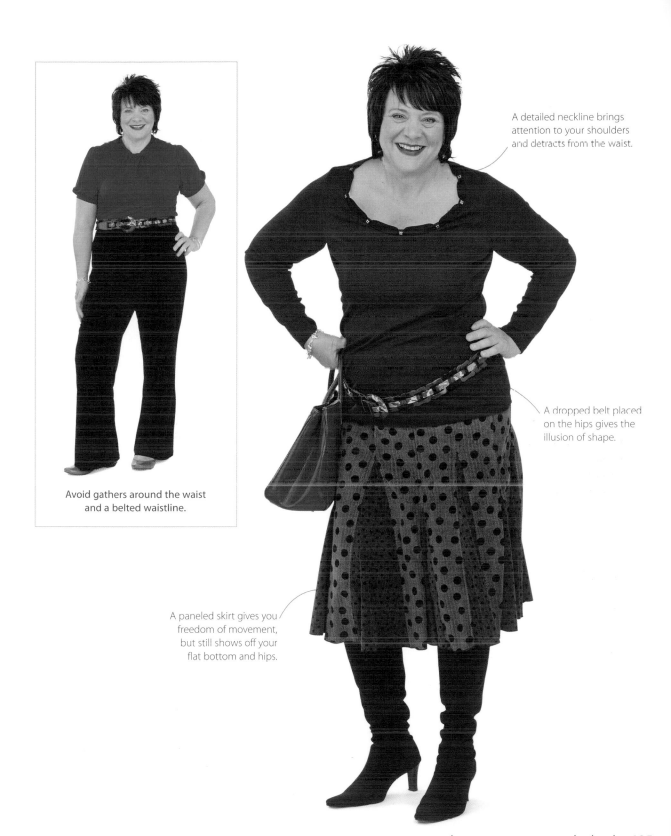

A detailed neckline brings attention to your shoulders and detracts from the waist.

A dropped belt placed on the hips gives the illusion of shape.

Avoid gathers around the waist and a belted waistline.

A paneled skirt gives you freedom of movement, but still shows off your flat bottom and hips.

# A younger **round** body

Make the most of the fact that you can wear loose, comfortable clothing lines. Long flowing lines will give you an elegant silhouette. Your fabrics need to be soft and fluid. Have the confidence to dress up these simple lines with fantastic accessories. Although the fabric may be soft, the clothing line needs to be straight. Bring attention to either the top third of your body or the lower third and avoid tucking your top in or belting.

## Shape basics
• You have a full bust.
• You have a full waist.
• You have soft facial features.

## What to wear

**Pants**  no waistband • drawstring • stretch waist • narrow • palazzo • flared

**Skirts**  no waistband • bias • knit • straight

**Tops**  caftan • wide T • loose shirt • gypsy

**Dresses**  A-line • shift • tunic and skirt

**Jackets**  deconstructed • long open-front • waterfall • swing • single-button collarless

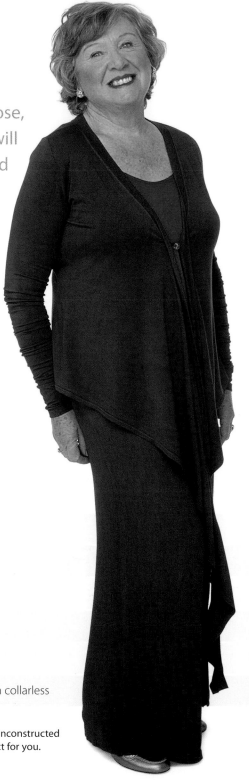

Loose-fitting, unconstructed lines are perfect for you.

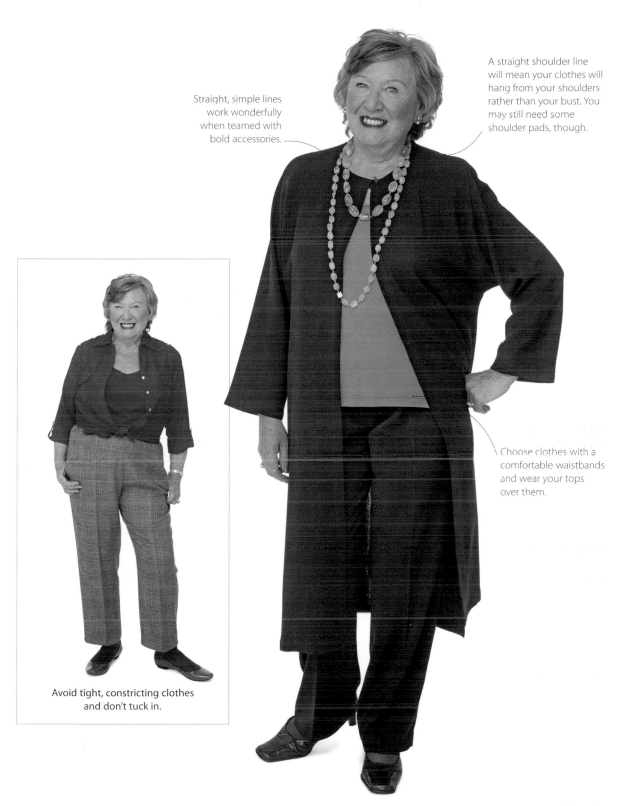

Straight, simple lines work wonderfully when teamed with bold accessories.

A straight shoulder line will mean your clothes will hang from your shoulders rather than your bust. You may still need some shoulder pads, though.

Choose clothes with a comfortable waistbands and wear your tops over them.

Avoid tight, constricting clothes and don't tuck in.

A younger round body **127**

# A question of size

Your scale—whether small, average, or large—will determine the size of pattern and the weight and texture of your clothes. Consider the following points in each case.

## Smaller scale

You may be short and have small bone structure and facial features. To look proportioned, and to ensure that your clothes don't overwhelm you, follow the suggestions below.

**Fabric textures:** Minimum texture, such as fine knits, pinwale corduroy, and lightweight tweed

**Fabric weight:** Lightweight, such as chiffon, lightweight wool, cotton lawn, and chambray

**Patterns:** Small

### Tips

• Dressing in one color from head to toe will make you look taller.

• Always wear fine jewelry.

• Keep hairstyles neat to balance your face.

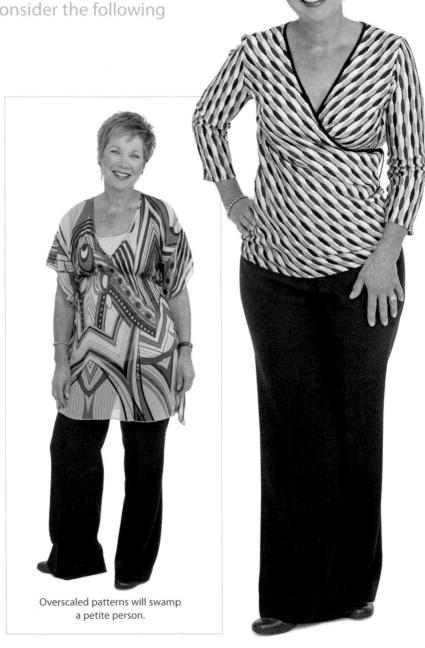

Overscaled patterns will swamp a petite person.

## Larger scale

You are likely to be taller than average, have overscale hands, feet, and facial features. To look balanced you need to wear clothes that reflect your heavier bone structure.

**Fabric textures:** Some texture, such as corduroy, tweed, and medium to heavy knits

**Fabric weight:** Medium- to heavyweight, such as raw silk, flannel, denim, and linen

**Patterns:** Medium to larger scale

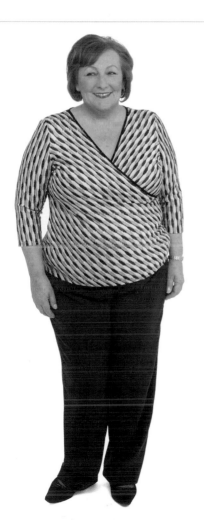

Small patterns don't balance with a grand-scaled woman, making her look larger.

### Tips

• If you are tall, break up your height using a different color.

• Wear larger-sized accessories.

• Fuller hairstyles balance your scale better.

• If you are an average size, you can do what you want… within reason!

# Good foundations

What you wear underneath your clothes is as important as your clothes themselves. Good foundations give you support, a good overall silhouette, and will control parts of your body that may need some holding back!

Intimate apparel is available in many colors (watch your palettes, ladies) and can be as plain or as sexy as you wish. Make sure you have a selection of suitable styles and colors to keep your underwear wardrobe young and stylish.

## Bras

A large proportion of women wear the wrong size bra. Over the years your bust will have changed shape and size and lost some of its firmness. Make sure to get yourself measured by an experienced corsetiere at least once a year. Be aware that there can be differences in sizing from one brand to another. And remember, the size of your bra doesn't matter, it's the fit that's important. The bust needs to be in the right place to get your clothes to fit properly.

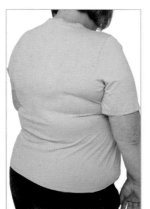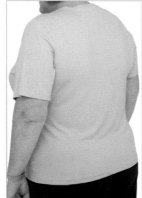

Your bra should not be seen through your clothes—if it is, it may be too small.

### Tips for fit

- The center of your bra should fit closely to the breastbone in order to lift and separate.

- There should be a smooth line where the fabric at the top of the cup ends and meets your bust. There should not be any ridges or bulging over the top or sides of the cups, even if you are wearing a balconette or lower-cut style.

- The strap around your body should be firm but comfortable, and it should be horizontal and not riding up at the back.

- Straps should not cut in or fall off the shoulders. If necessary, choose a style with a wider strap (particularly if you have a large bust).

Ideally you should have a selection of bra styles to suit the different types of top you tend to wear. For example, the bra you will wear under a T-shirt will be a different one from the one you wear under an evening top. Your bra should never be visible through your top.

### Bra styles
**Bra tops:** The cups are part of a T-shirt. These are for the small-chested only.
**T-shirt/seamless:** These give a cleaner line underneath tight clothing and lightweight fabrics.

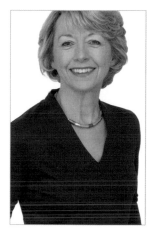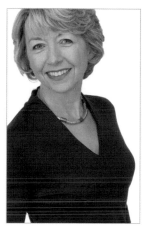

A small bust can easily be enhanced with insets or a padded bra.

**Sports:** These give good support to the bust and are designed to reduce breast bounce.

**Nonwired/soft:** If you have a large back, it will be easier to find a better fit with a nonwired bra than with an underwired one.

**Underwired:** These offer added support and shape and minimize sagging. This is the most versatile style for most women.

**Balconette:** A low neckline goes straight across the bust with wide-set straps for a square neckline. These are suitable for wearing with lower-cut tops.

**Full-cup bra:** This covers the entire breast and is designed to give full support.

**Minimizer:** This redistributes the breast so that it does not protrude as much. These are good for wearing under a shirt.

**Push-up:** This lifts the bust up and enhances the cleavage. Not for the work environment!

**Padded:** These enhance a small bust and can give it a slight lift. They come with removable pads.

## Panties

Your choice of panties will depend on your size, the comfort you are seeking, the shape and firmness of your bottom, and what you are wearing. Make sure there is no "visible panty line" (VPL) and that the color of your panties coordinates with what you are wearing. It is often better to buy panties a size larger, in case they shrink in the wash.

### Panty styles

**Thong/g-string:** These offer the traditional way to banish the VPL, and leave the bottom bare; only for a slim, pert bottom.

**Brief:** The waistband sits on or just below the belly button and gives full side and back coverage. They are best for firm, pert bottoms that don't need any control.

**"Boyshorts"/boxers:** These are like briefs, but with a lower-cut leg that finishes at the top of the leg rather than across the bottom. These are good for avoiding VPL and certainly more comfortable than thongs for large bottoms.

**Tap pants:** These are a comfortable, loose, feminine cut with no control. Perfect under full skirts and dresses.

**High leg:** This is a brief with a cutaway leg that gives the illusion of a longer leg.

**Bikini:** Here, the top of the panties sits on the hip line. They can be either high or low leg.

**Tummy control:** These are available in different styles, from brief to full panties, and with a front panel in stretch fabric to shape and support the tummy and bottom.

**Smoothers or "power panties":** These garments can control the thighs, lift the bottom, flatten the tummy, and give you a waist. Make sure you can breathe when wearing them!

### Going one step further

- An "all-in-one" will support and enhance your bust, while flattening your stomach and firming the bottom. This is a great choice for when you want a smooth silhouette.

- "Control-top panty hose" have a top section offering allover control for a little toning.

# Fine-tuning your wardrobe

A closet full of clutter is impossible to manage and hard to use effectively. You may well have collected a host of fashion items over the years and are probably clinging to them in the hope that they will come back in.

Take some advice and get rid of them! Even if the same shape, color, or fabric were to become fashionable again, it would always be different, however slightly, from what you have been hoarding. And there is nothing that will date you quicker than wearing yesteryear's statement pieces. So if you are the kind of woman that has an obsession with collecting bags, shoes, white tops, or black trousers, some serious fine-tuning is called for.

A great time to sort out your closet is when the weather changes and you switch over from cold-weather to warm-weather clothes. Take each item in turn and ask yourself whether or not you have

## Tips

- Don't keep any items simply for best; by the time you get around to wearing them, they'll probably be out of date.

- If anything has passed its sell-by-date (in particular shoes), get rid of it.

- Do you know what you have gathering dust on the top shelf of your wardrobe? Now is the time to clear it out.

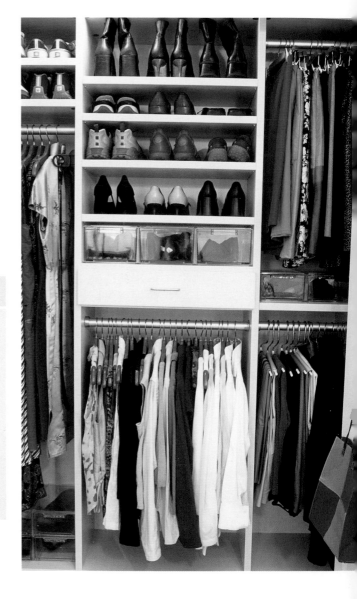

A well-organized wardrobe makes dressing each day easier as you can see what you have available.

worn it in the past six months. If the answer is no, and you are about to store it for another six months, ask yourself again whether you really need to keep it.

Organize your closet in groups of clothes. Put all your jackets together, then your skirts, then your pants, and so on. Even if you have purchased garments as suits, split them up to give you more options to mix and match. Work on the concept of fewer clothes but more options to wear.

## The core wardrobe

This is a basic guideline of what you might want to have in your wardrobe in your 40s, 50s, 60s, and beyond. You may be juggling a job and family, or enjoying a little more free time (and even a little more money to spend on yourself). Or perhaps you are considering a complete change of lifestyle…

The chart below shows you how many of each piece you need to jump-start a wardrobe that will take you from a casual to a more formal look.

| Clothing | In your 40s | In your 50s | In your 60s and beyond |
| --- | --- | --- | --- |
| Formal pants | 3 | 3 | 2 |
| Casual pants | 3 | 3 | 4 |
| Jeans | 2 | 1 | 1 |
| Formal skirts | 2 | 3 | 2 |
| Casual skirts | 2 | 3 | 3 |
| T-shirts | 6 | 5 | 5 |
| Shirts/blouses | 4 | 4 | 4 |
| Sweaters (knitwear) | 6 | 8 | 6 |
| Cardigans | 2 | 3 | 3 |
| Day dresses | 2 | 3 | 2 |
| Casual dresses (including summer) | 4 | 5 | 6 |
| Party dresses | 2 | 3 | 4 |
| Formal jackets | 4 | 3 | 2 |
| Coats | 1 | 1 | 1 |
| Casual outerwear | 1 | 2 | 3 |

# How to shop

You are already aware that, while a garment from one store in a certain size will fit you, a similar garment in the same size from another store will fit either differently or not at all.

This knowledge may not make you feel any better about yourself, but has to be accepted as one of the challenges you face in seeking a younger-looking you. What you have to remember is that getting the right fit is crucial to achieving your goal. If it means buying a bigger size, or a different cut or fabric, it is time to face up to it. The key with any item of clothing is that there is enough ease to allow you to move around comfortably, but not so much that you look swamped.

## Things to keep in mind

When trying on clothes, it is better to wear a complete outfit instead of trying pieces in isolation. For example, a smart suit will not look its best if tried on with a T-shirt and sneakers. Take the right top and shoes with you; make sure your underwear is neutral in color and won't give you a VPL, especially if you intend to try on pale colors.

Not all store mirrors are the same, and some can distort the way you look back at yourself. The lighting in a store might affect the color of a garment, too, and it is a good idea to check the look of an outfit in natural daylight if you can.

## Getting the right fit

### Skirts
• For a pencil skirt, you should be able to easily pinch about 1 inch (2.5 cm) of fabric at your hip when standing.
• Stop the skirt hem at a point on your leg where it narrows, usually just below the knee or lower calf

to ankle (this rule also applies to cropped pants).
• When trying on a straight skirt, make sure you can sit down comfortably without the skirt riding up. If it does, try on another style in a different fabric.

### Pants
• You should be able to get a couple of fingers comfortably under the waistband without having to breathe in.
• Any side pockets should lie flat; if they are bulging, try the next size up or a different style.
• Wide-leg pants should be long enough to cover the foot at the front and fall over the shoe and heel at the back. Make sure they are not too long, or you will trip over.
• Narrow-leg pants should not fall over the shoe. To get a perfect fit, the hem of the pants may need to slant from front to back.

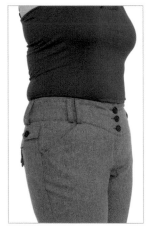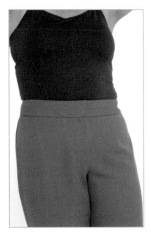

You need flat hips and bottom to wear pants with details (left), otherwise go for plain designs (right).

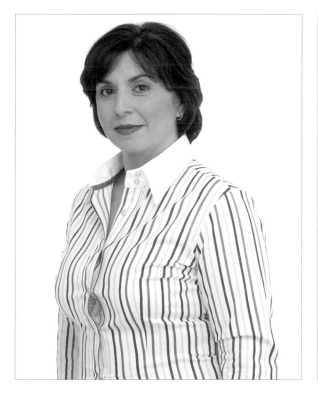

Shirts in crisp fabrics don't work on a full bust and will never fit properly, as shown above.

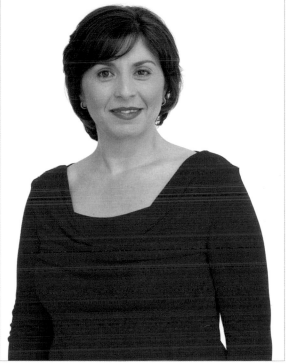

A top in soft fabric with no front opening is flattering over the bust, and to the neckline.

## Shirts
• Front buttons should not gape.
• Allow for movement across the shoulders.
• A set-in sleeve should sit at the edge of your shoulders and hang straight.

## Sleeves
• Long sleeves should finish just below or on your wrist bone.
• Short sleeves should finish at a narrow point on your arm.
• Sleeves should not be tight over the upper arm.

## Coats
• Make sure your coat is at least 1 inch (2.5 cm) longer than your skirt.
• Always try winter coats on over what you will be wearing underneath.

• A coat needs to fasten comfortably and should not pull around the bust, pockets, or buttons. Make sure the neckline flatters your neck length.

### Tips

• When you find a clothing brand that fits you well, go back to it for more.

• The true cost of a garment is not what you pay for it, but how often you wear it. Sometimes the more expensive item that you wear many times over is a much better buy than the bargain you wear only once or twice.

# Body perfect

Many a woman feels that her body is far from perfect. If you fall into this category, rest assured that there are plenty of ways of dealing with those parts that you feel you must hide.

In many cases, it is not actually a matter of hiding them but, rather, dressing them correctly. Often, this can be as simple as taking the eye away from the "offending" area in order to give the illusion of a perfect feature.

## Your neck

Q: How can I make my neck look longer?
A: Keep your neckline open (V-necks and scoops are best) and avoid clutter.

Q: I think my neck is thick—what do I do?
A: Keep your hair short and do not clutter the neck area by wearing chokers. Don't knot a scarf around your neck.

Q: What do I do with my long neck?
A: You can wear high collars (turtlenecks,

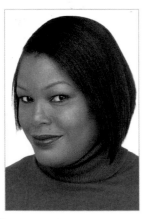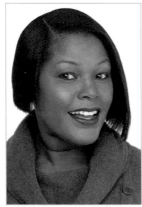

A short neck needs a dropped collar or open neckline, which help make the neck appear longer.

mandarin) and add details (chokers and scarves are great on you). Long hair will work well too.

## Your shoulders

Q: How can I make my shoulders appear bigger?
A: Try building them up by adding small, soft shoulder pads. Wear straight-seam shirts with set-in sleeves rather than raglan.

## Your décolleté (from neck to cleavage)

Q: What can I wear in the evening? I do not wear low necklines because I feel my décolleté is lined.
A: Think about wearing a chiffon top or hide it with necklaces; don't forget to use your sunblock from now on.

## Your chest

Q: I have no boobs to speak of, so why should I wear a bra?
A: A correctly fitted bra will give you some shape; even small breasts need support for a feminine silhouette. Try adding details and texture in fabrics to your tops.

Q: How do I minimize my big boobs?
A: Go to a specialized lingerie shop and be professionally measured. Then, avoid details (pockets, embroidery, buttons) over the bust. A wrap top is more accommodating than anything that is front-opening. Don't wear sleeves that finish in line with the fullest part of your bust. Avoid carrying a bag high underneath your arm.

## Your waist

Q: Can I wear a belt? My waist seems to have gotten thicker.
A: If you still have a defined, feminine waist, of course you can wear a belt. Make sure its scale is appropriate for you.

Q: Why is it that I do not like to tuck in anymore?
A: There may be very little space between your waist and your bust (your bust may have increased in size) and you have the appearance of being slightly short-waisted. Try lowering your waistline (no waistband on skirts and pants) and not tucking in. Wearing a belt below the natural waistline will also give the illusion of a lower waist.

## Your tummy

Q: What can I do to hide my tummy, which has not gone away since I had my children?
A: Your rounded tummy is a mark of being female. Don't be fanatical about trying to achieve a flat stomach; that is the prerogative of men. Avoid details that add volume (front zippers, front patch pockets, open pleats). Instead, go for flat-fronted trousers and skirts. Patterns (not stripes and checks) will also help to disguise your tummy, as will wearing a dropped belt. A looser fit will be more flattering.

## Your bum

Q: Why is it that pants never seem to come up to my waist?
A: This is because you have a long bottom. By selecting drop-waist pants (and skirts) you will get a better fit. To break up this area, try layering your tops.

Q: What can I do to hide my sticking-out butt?
A: Try wearing tops and jackets with peplums, which are great for fitting over this area. Skirts and pants with darts going into the waistband also work well with this type of bottom.

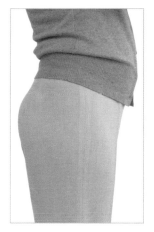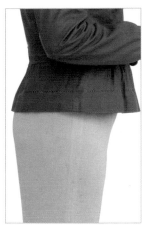

A good way to disguise a full bottom is to wear a waisted top or peplum.

Q: Can I still wear jeans? They seem to make my butt look huge.
A: Yes you can, but avoid jeans with lots of details on your bottom, such as pockets, appliqués, and branding. Bootleg and wide-leg styles are more flattering than tapered ones. A stretch denim (in a darker shade) will also accommodate your curved hips and bottom.

## Your hips

Q: Can I wear a short top? My hips are huge, and I usually hide them underneath a big top.
A: Yes, you can. Swamping yourself into a big top only makes things worse. Draw attention to the upper part of your body with pattern, texture, and accessories. If you have a waist, you can tuck in. If not, your top needs to finish just below your waistline and above your widest part.

## Your thighs

Q: What can I do about my thighs?
A: You can wear wide-leg, loose pants; skirts and pants need to hang straight and not "hug" your bottom or curve underneath. Fabrics are better when softer and more fluid rather than stiff.

# A younger
# look

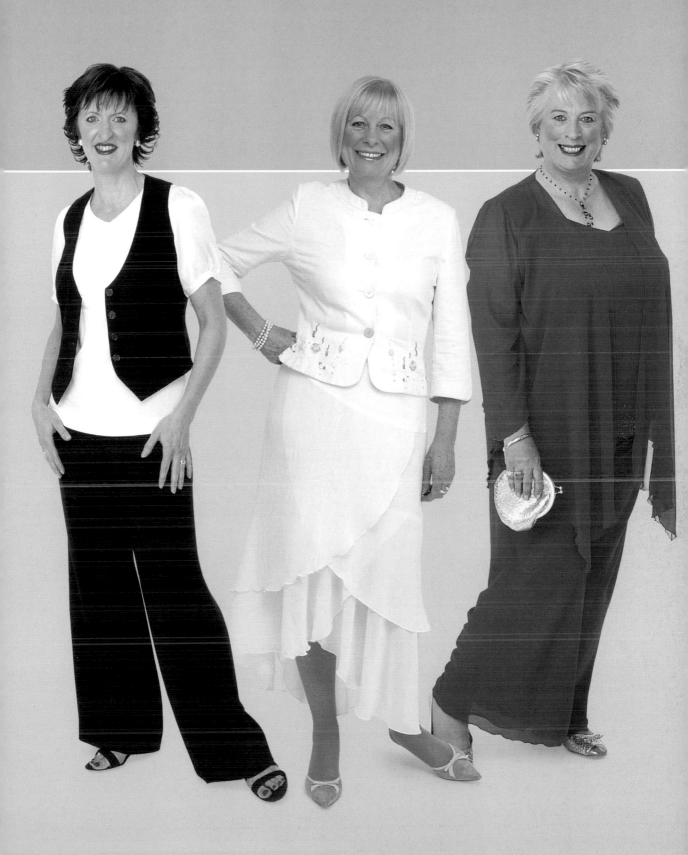

# Your style

Your personal preferences will determine the types of clothes you like to wear, feel most comfortable in, and that are appropriate for your lifestyle. By adapting these preferences, and by moving with the prevalent trends, you can stay looking younger for longer.

To help you make informed decisions about what you should wear, you need to determine and understand your style personality. Once you establish this, you'll see why you prefer to wear a pair of loafers to spike heels.

Fill in the following questionnaire, checking the answers that best describe you, and it will all fall into place.

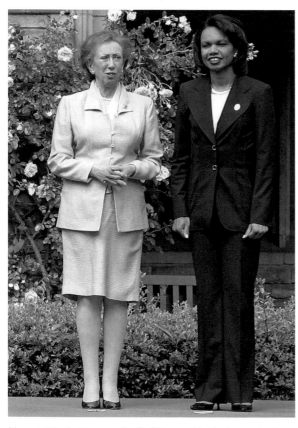

Margaret Beckett wears a badly fitting suit in the inappropriate color of baby pink, while Condoleezza Rice appears well groomed in her appropriately colored, businesslike suit.

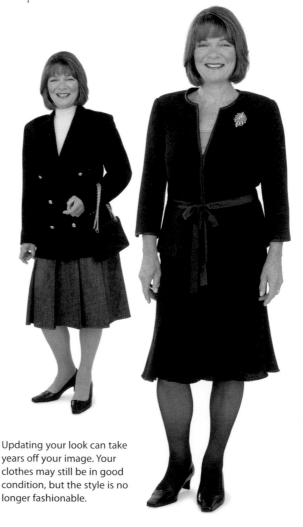

Updating your look can take years off your image. Your clothes may still be in good condition, but the style is no longer fashionable.

## Your hair

**a** I love to put accessories in my hair.

**b** I'm always changing the color of my hair.

**c** I like to keep it long.

**d** It has to be styled and neat.

**e** It needs to be easy to maintain.

**f** I take my hairdresser's advice.

## Your tops

**a** I get mine anywhere, including thrift shops and bazaars.

**b** I buy one every week.

**c** I like details on mine.

**d** I like a neat blouse or shirt.

**e** They need to be comfortable and washable.

**f** I like simple styles.

## Your dream vacations

**a** Traveling around Southeast Asia.

**b** Skiing in Aspen.

**c** A weekend in Paris with someone special.

**d** A cruise.

**e** A safari.

**f** Visiting art galleries in London or Florence.

## Your jeans

**a** I like vintage ones.

**b** I like designer jeans.

**c** I wear them sometimes, but prefer skirts.

**d** I don't own a pair.

**e** I wear them all the time.

**f** I like smart ones.

## Your bags

**a** I like tapestry and fabric bags.

**b** The bolder, the better.

**c** I change my bag all the time to match my outfit.

**d** Mine matches my shoes.

**e** I have to get everything into it.

**f** It has to be the current shape and color.

Count how many a, b, c, etc. answers you have.

Mainly **a**    you are a **creative** (see page 142)

Mainly **b**    you are a **dramatic** (see page 143)

Mainly **c**    you are a **romantic** (see page 144)

Mainly **d**    you are a **classic** (see page 145)

Mainly **e**    you are a **natural** (see page 146)

Mainly **f**    you are a **city chic** (see page 147)

If you have a mixture of answers, this could mean that your wardrobe needs careful investigation! It may mean that, because your lifestyle is changing, you are in transition and trying to find yourself. Read the relevant pages and see which style you feel most comfortable with.

# The creative

If this is you, you take pride in originating a look to suit your personality. You love shopping and revel in rummaging through secondhand stores for vintage classics to team with your latest fashion purchases.

## Style traits
• You have a unique look.
• You dislike a coordinated and packaged look.
• You have creative hobbies, such as drawing, painting, and writing.

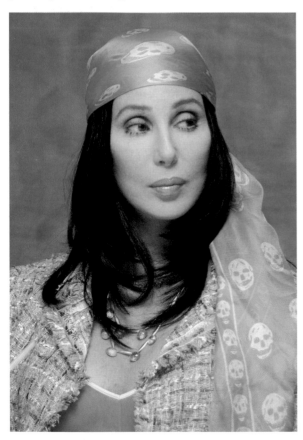
Cher mixes couture clothes with cheerful accessories for an upbeat and creative look.

## Your wardrobe **in your 40s**
• Start wearing makeup for a more groomed look.
• Keep your clothes well maintained.
• Make sure that your top and bottom color combinations work well together and are in your right colors.
• If you have kept your funky boots, you can still wear them with your evening look.
• Find an unusual vintage coat for day or night.

## Your wardrobe **in your 50s**
• Keep in mind that colorful highlights and extensions in your hair will look more youthful than a crazy block color.
• Don't hide your body in long, voluminous layers.
• Replace the knitted hat with a felt one.
• Go wild with shoes and boots.
• Indulge in some printed fabrics or fake-fur shoes and bags.

## Your wardrobe **in your 60s and beyond**
• Try to avoid looking like an aging hippie. You have developed your own style, but you may need to keep it under control.
• Keep your hair shorter and more manageable, but add an interesting color.
• Mix textures and fabrics, but keep the colors of these clothes the same.
• Go for ethnic accessories when wearing simple or plain tops.
• Shop when you travel to keep your unique look.

# The dramatic

If this is you, you buy clothes that you know will turn a few heads. You are something of an impulse buyer, are drawn to the latest fashions, and have to shop and read fashion magazines in order to keep up to date.

## Style traits
• You like to be noticed for what you wear.
• You like bold contrasting colors, often worn with black.
• You get a buzz out of your hobbies.

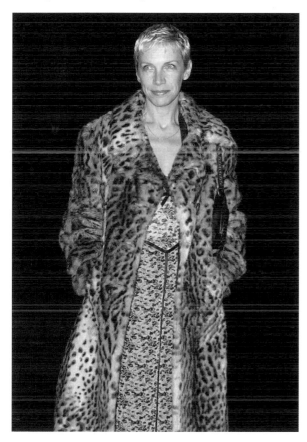

Annie Lennox combines dramatic individual pieces for a stunning look.

## Your wardrobe **in your 40s**
• Showing your cleavage is fine, but not your midriff or tummy.
• Use brightly patterned tops and contrasting color to give drama to your look.
• If you have the figure, embellish your jeans and wear them with cowboy boots.
• Indulge in a few statement accessories.
• Wear a white dress for an evening function to guarantee that you make an entrance.

## Your wardrobe **in your 50s**
• If black is not in your palette, use high contrast and the brighter colors of your palette.
• Keep your animal prints to one garment to keep your look age appropriate.
• For your casual look, wear a big white shirt buttoned or unbuttoned, depending on your figure.
• Make sure your jackets have some trim details.
• Wear big sunglasses for the wow factor.

## Your wardrobe **in your 60s and beyond**
• Put some red in your wardrobe for an energizing boost and emotional lift.
• Use statement accessories for a young and glamorous look.
• Add a vest to your shirts and blouses.
• Try plain bootleg jeans and a heeled ankle boot for a youthful way of wearing pants.
• Either wear a colorful hat, scarf, or gloves with your winter coat, or make your coat a colorful one.

# The romantic

If this is you, you are seduced by any item of clothing with detail —frills, flounces, and fringes abound in your wardrobe. You love looking and feeling feminine and airy and invariably choose pretty fabrics.

## Style traits
• You love luxurious, textured fabrics.
• You wear pink with a flourish.
• You are a spectator of, rather than a participant in, any form of sports.

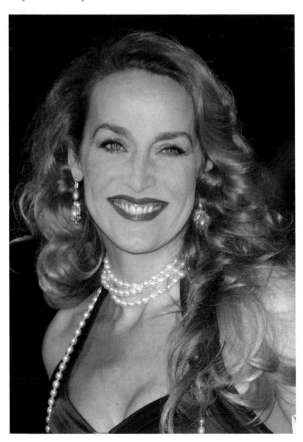

Jerry Hall has managed to keep her beautiful and romantic image as she matures.

## Your wardrobe **in your 40s**
• Turn your frills into flounces, and ribbon details into bows.
• For a working environment, mix your pinks with medium to dark neutral colors.
• You might find that a waisted jacket with a peplum works for you.
• Look for skirts with some movement and kick to the hemline.
• If you hair is long and layered, don't detract from it by wearing too much detailed jewelry.

## Your wardrobe **in your 50s**
• Find a shoulder-length hairstyle that you like.
• Add chiffon and lace to your tops.
• Wear long floral dresses with wedge or strappy sandals.
• Accessorize your legs with pretty patterned stockings or tights.
• Go for a patterned winter coat to give you a younger look.

## Your wardrobe **in your 60s and beyond**
• Keep your florals for scarves and bags.
• Make sure that your more sensible underwear is still pretty.
• Use barrettes or clips in your hair rather than flowers and ribbons.
• Try fake-fur trims on cardigans and coats.
• Abandon your spike heels and go for a stacked or kitten heel instead.

# The classic

If this is you, you are most comfortable in timeless, established styles that give you the elegant yet formal appearance you favor. Your look is essentially well coordinated and you rarely dabble with bold colors or striking patterns.

## Style traits
- You have the most coordinated wardrobe of all the personalities.
- You plan your shopping trips.
- You are an accomplished homemaker.

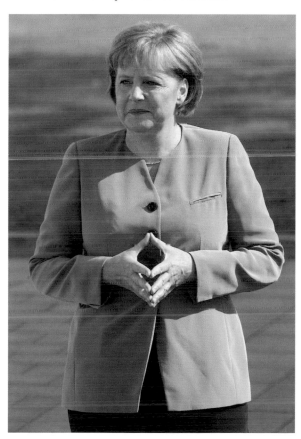

Angela Merkel is always well turned out and efficient looking, as befits her position as German chancellor.

## Your wardrobe **in your 40s**
- Replace the blazer with an updated jacket style.
- Choose a fitted shirt to suit your body shape.
- For a makeover, try a wrap dress or top over a pair of pants.
- Add new costume jewelry to your existing jewelry in the evening.
- Try carrying a fun bag rather than your usual investment one.

## Your wardrobe **in your 50s**
- Enjoy your twinset, but load up the pearls.
- Nothing dates you more than your hairstyle, so update your look.
- Change your winter coat for an ageless style.
- If you choose to wear stretch waistbands, make sure they don't show.
- Buy your shoes in good chain stores.

## Your wardrobe **in your 60s and beyond**
- If you have not done so already, change your hair color and style.
- Now that you may have a little more time, read some fashion magazines to keep abreast of trends.
- Instead of throwing out your suits, wear the jackets and skirts separately with more casual pieces.
- Denim may not be your favorite, but try linen or chambray for a more relaxed and youthful look.
- Break the matching-shoes and-bag rule and enjoy the difference.

# The natural

If this is you, you are not one for fuss and frippery. Comfort is your priority when it comes to shopping for clothes, and you prefer a simple but casual look, with the bare minimum of added accessories.

## Style traits
• You have a relaxed attitude to dressing.
• You feel most comfortable in dress-down and (business) casual.
• You enjoy walking, gardening, and pets.

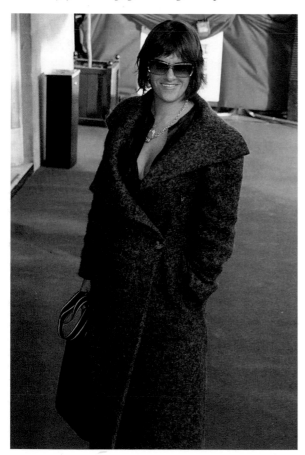

Artist Tracey Emin loves her comfortable sneakers and big roomy coat, while sunglasses hide the lack of makeup.

## Your wardrobe **in your 40s**
• If your lifestyle calls for a suit, make it a fashionable pantsuit.
• Stick to wearing T-shirts and knitwear instead of shirts and blouses.
• For comfort, buy a long skirt rather than a short, straight one.
• Consider a long cardigan to double up as a coat.
• Flats are comfortable, but consider a kitten heel for a younger look.

## Your wardrobe **in your 50s**
• Buy easy-to-wear pants in stretch fabrics, so that you can still sit on the floor.
• Have fun layering shirts and T-shirts.
• Wear dresses long in an easy fit, with a pair of colorful pumps or ballet flats.
• Go for fashionable and fun waterproofs for your outdoor activities.
• Buy fashionable sneakers in neutral colors to complement your relaxed style.

## Your wardrobe **in your 60s and beyond**
• Knitwear for all occasions is a comfortable winner all year round.
• Try a long wrap skirt for a fashionable, comfortable, and young look.
• Wear a shirt as a deconstructed jacket.
• Think of bringing in a denim skirt to replace your favorite jeans.
• Keep your shoes and boots modern and make sure they are appropriate for the rest of your outfit.

# The city chic

If this is you, you favor a look that relies on established trends rather than fleeting fashions. You like to have a coordinated look, wearing colors tone-on-tone rather than contrasting bold with neutral.

## Style traits
- You always have the right outfit to wear for any type of occasion.
- You feel comfortable in both your formal and casual clothes.
- Pastimes and hobbies are organized and social.

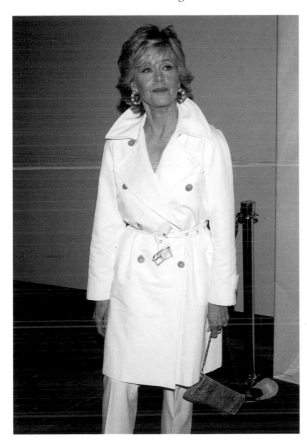

Jane Fonda wears a classic trench coat and slacks, but has updated her accessories.

## Your wardrobe **in your 40s**
- Don't give up on fashion for your workwear.
- Mix shirts and knitwear for a young look.
- Wear your jeans with a suit jacket for a different, fun look.
- Buy a knee-length coat as a great addition to your wardrobe.
- Introduce color to your tops, especially for summertime or your vacation wardrobe.

## Your wardrobe **in your 50s**
- Investigate new stores and labels that you feel comfortable in.
- Add some patterns or details to your tops.
- Buy deconstructed jackets to give you a softer-looking silhouette.
- Add a pair of cropped pants with boots or flats for a younger look.
- Forget your investment shoes, and go for fun and funky styles.

## Your wardrobe **in your 60s and beyond**
- Create an an elegant and youthful look with bias-cut dresses—long or short.
- Make your casual wardrobe your core wardrobe now, and concentrate your investment here.
- Try replacing your jacket with a beautiful knitted cardigan in your colors.
- Make your raincoat colorful to cheer up those dank, rainy days.
- Keep your costume jewelry updated with some fun pieces.

# Accessories

Now that you know what to wear to give you a younger look, make sure you do not spoil the effect with the wrong or outdated accessories. Often, the accessories alone will update an existing outfit. It just needs a little thought.

## Panty hose, thigh-highs, stockings, knee-highs

Keep wearing stockings (with a garter belt) or thigh-highs as long as they are comfortable. Thigh-highs are good in hot weather if you need to have a formal look or to cover your legs. Panty hose with gentle control are great for helping tighten around your tummy. When selecting knee-highs, watch out for tight bands that might restrict the circulation under the knee: select as wide a band as you can.

## Whether or not to go bare legged

To go bare legged you need to have toned, unblemished legs. Consider using a fake tan. Unfortunately, if you have varicose veins, only wear long skirts or pants if you wish to be bare legged in the summer.

## Shoes

The degree to which you match the style of the shoes you wear with your clothes will be key to your looking young and trendy. Formalwear needs formal shoes; casualwear needs casual shoes, and so on. When it comes to the height of the heel, the general rule is that the shorter the skirt, the lower the heel. This is because a short skirt and a high heel are not balanced and have the effect of elongating the leg, making it look out of proportion with the length of the skirt.

Shoes are a girl's best friend. Buy them, wear them, and change them every day.

> ### Tips
>
> - **In winter:** Tone the color of your panty hose with the color of your dress/skirt/pants and ditch the "tan"-colored hose.
>
> - **In summer:** Low-denier, flesh-colored, hose are best, with sheer toes.

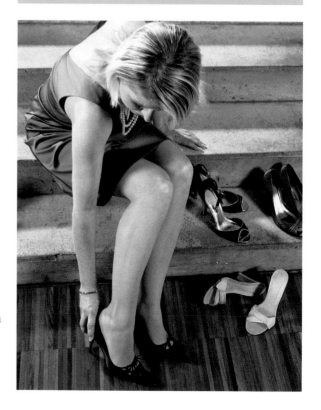

| Shoe type | Wear with | Leg wear |
|---|---|---|
| Loafers | Pants and jeans; winter skirts | Socks or knee-highs; opaque tights; patterned tights |
| High front; low heel | Pants; skirts (if long legged and slim ankled) | Socks or knee-highs; opaque tights (in winter); sheer hose (in summer) |
| Heeled pump | Skirts and dresses; formal pants | Sheer or opaque tights in winter; patterned knee-highs |
| Spike heels | Dresses | Sheer hose; bare legs |
| T-strap (If good ankles): | Skirts; dresses | Sheer or opaque hose, depending on weight of shoes and clothes |
| Mules | Pants; skirts and dresses | Bare legs in hot weather |
| Ballet flats | In the summer with: pants, jeans, skirts, dresses. In the winter with: evening pants | Bare in the summer; sheer knee-highs in winter |
| Flat sandals | Pants and jeans; skirts and dresses | Bare legs |
| Heeled strappy sandals | Skirts and dresses | Bare legs |

| Boot type | Wear with |
|---|---|
| Chelsea | Pants and jeans |
| Flat, loose calf boot | Pants (tucked in); skirts |
| Heeled ankle boot | Pants; long skirts |
| Flat knee-high | Pants and jeans; skirts |
| Medium-heel knee-high | Pants and jeans; skirts and dresses |
| Heeled boot | Pants and jeans; skirts and dresses |

**Tips**

- If you are wearing boots with pants and jeans, socks and knee-highs are best.

- Make sure your boots end at a slim part of your legs: anything finishing at a wide point of the leg (and this includes your hemline) only emphasizes the width of the leg at that point.

## Costume jewelry

Costume jewelry is a great way of keeping your look youthful; be bold enough to mix it with your investment pieces. There are a few things you need to consider when buying jewelry. Don't be afraid of mixing real with fake. Adding jewelry to your daytime wardrobe is all it needs to take you to an evening look.

### What to look for

**Color:** The colors should complement or contrast with the colors that you wear. Often, a darker color from your palette will look striking with a lighter-colored necklace (for example, light beads or pearls with a black or navy top). If you are wearing neutral colors from your palette, team them either with light- or fashion-colored jewelry.

**Scale:** Consider your bone structure when selecting pieces and make sure that your jewelry doesn't overwhelm you if you are on the small side, or get lost if you are large. If you are petite, only one large statement piece will work (either a necklace or a pin, but not both together). If you are grand scale, lots of lightweight pieces can work very well together.

**Face shapes:** Try to counterbalance the shape of your face with the shape of your jewelry. For example, angled face shapes need softening and can wear rounder-shaped earrings, while softer, more rounded faces will benefit from a few angles.

**Proportions:** Consider your neck when choosing earrings and necklaces.

For a long neck, you should look out for chokers, multiple-strand necklaces and long earrings. Longer-length necklaces and shorter earrings are more suitable if you have a short neck.

**Chest and cleavage:** Adding necklaces and brooches or pins will enhance a small bust. If you expose your cleavage, make sure your pendant doesn't dangle in it or sit on it. Above or below the chest is where your jewelry should sit.

**Arms and hands:** Whether you decide to wear a single bracelet or lots of them is a personal choice, but if you have short arms do not overload your wrist to the extreme. If you have long arms you can pile on as many bracelets as you want. Always wear rings—costume or the real thing—that balance the scale of your hand.

### Tip

• Don't forget that watches and glasses are accessories too. In both cases, you need to think about color, style, and scale. You may want to consider having a selection of watches and a couple of pairs of glasses for different occasions.

A simple dress is made to look fantastic with the addition of a necklace, shoes, and bag.

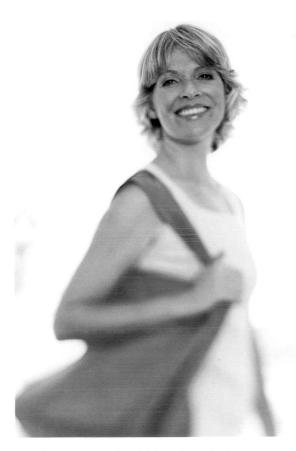

When buying accessories, pick items in a color from your palette to make sure it works for you.

## It's in the bag

Bags, like shoes, will date your look. You need to have a small selection of bags to suit different occasions and what you wear. To stay young and fashionable, you need to consider adding to your selection, and this can now be done without breaking the bank.

Choosing a bag is a very personal thing. You need to think of the practicalities. If you need to be hands-free you may like a backpack, or long-handled/-strapped bag. If not, a handbag or clutch bag will be fine.

Sometimes you need a large, practical bag to carry everything from a spare pair of shoes to a laptop. Have a smaller, more manageable bag inside, to go off to lunch or the theater.

### What to look for
**Color:** For an all-purpose day bag, choose a neutral color from your palette. It does not have to be black, brown, or navy, nor does it have to match your shoes.

**Size and shape:** Consider what you need to put in it, and then your scale and body lines. Make sure, by looking in a mirror, that the bag balances with your silhouette.

**Occasion bags:** Think about the practicalities of the bag.

## Scarves
The quickest way to update your look and add color to an outfit is with a scarf.

### What to look for
**Color:** A scarf is the ideal way to introduce color to your wardrobe either in contrast to what you are wearing or as part of a tone-on-tone outfit.

**Size:** Small women should seek out small, plain scarves or those with a dainty pattern. Larger-scale women can wearer bolder scarves, both in pattern and size.

**Fabric:** Consider the weight of the fabric: a heavy-knit scarf will dwarf a petite woman, who should choose scarves that are made from lightweight fabrics instead.

**Style:** Consider your neck length when wearing a scarf. A bulky knot around a short or wide neck will not be as flattering as wearing it loose. If you have a long neck, you can use a scarf to accessorize your neckline.

# Party time

What fun! You've been invited to a party, a wedding, or a special event. After the initial euphoria, panic sets in. Too late, you have accepted and Cinderella will have to go to the ball!

## Questions to ask yourself
• Is the party indoors or outdoors?
• Is it a sitting or standing occasion?
• Is it during the day or evening?
• Will it be glamorous or relaxed?
• Do you want to steal the show or play it down?

By answering these questions, you will be able to decide on an appropriate outfit in which you can look young and stylish. At all times, refer to your color palette, your body shape, scale, proportion, and style personality. Get it right and you will look like a million dollars.

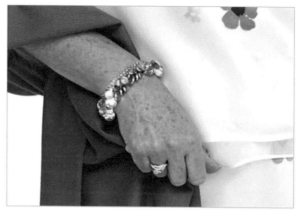

Sparkling accessories can change the look of a daytime outfit and make it special for party time.

## Tips

• Be wary of the advice you may get in a store if you announce that you are looking for a "special event" outfit. You may leave with a head-to-toe matching outfit that you'll never wear again.

• Always try things on before rejecting them.

• Think about whether you have anything in your wardrobe that you can add to and accessorize.

• If you want to enjoy the event, make sure that you are comfortable in what you wear, including underwear and shoes.

• Think about how you might possibly wear the outfit again, either all together or separated and mixed with other garments.

• When it comes to accessories, beads and appliqués on knits are ageless.

• Remember that patterns and soft layering of beaded chiffon can hide a multitude of sins.

• Use purples, teals, medium blues, and reds as alternatives to black.

• Remember that beaded accessories can add glamour to an evening look.

• Spend a little more time and effort applying your makeup—it will pay dividends because it will stay on longer.

## Partying **in your 40s**

• Keep wearing your strappy tops and dresses as long as you feel comfortable in them.

• Make sure that the volume of your evening wear doesn't overwhelm your scale.

• Don't shy away from having fun with strong colors, as long as they are in your palette.

• Consider purchasing a fantastic evening pantsuit (tuxedo), which is a great investment buy and could last for years. This can be dressed up with a bustier, a strappy shell, a sequin top, or nothing (if you button the jacket!).

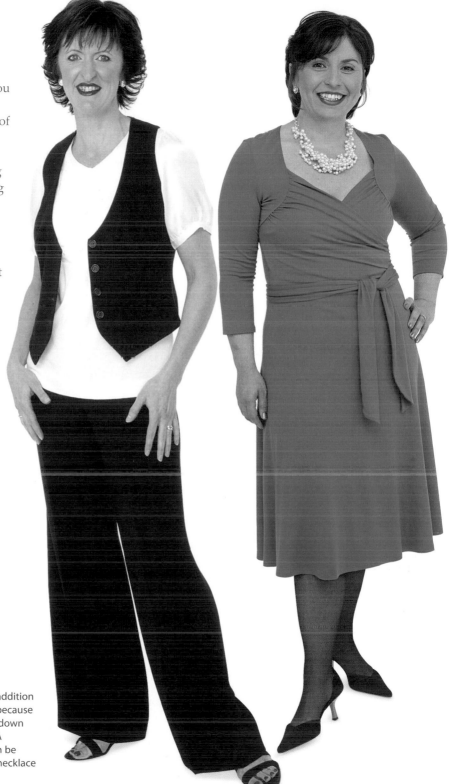

Fun separates are a great addition to your formal wardrobe, because you can dress them up or down depending on the event. A fabulous-colored dress can be accessorized with a great necklace and evening shoes.

## Partying **in your 50s**

• If you are concerned about showing too much flesh, a slit skirt is a fun way to remain young and sexy.

• If black is not in your palette, add metallics and shimmering fabrics.

• Try a long, slender, silk dress for evening glamour.

• If making an investment buy, consider a beaded or sequined jacket that you can wear with your little black dress, with evening pants, or with a long or short skirt.

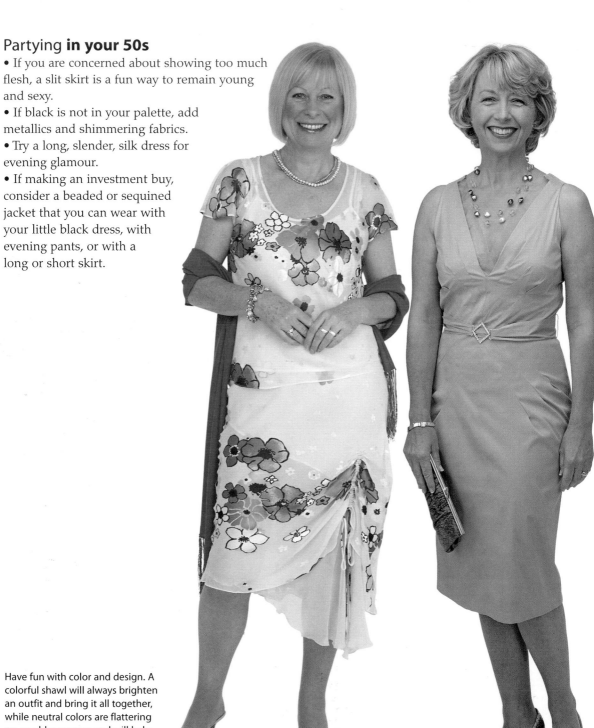

Have fun with color and design. A colorful shawl will always brighten an outfit and bring it all together, while neutral colors are flattering on an older woman and will help her stand out in a room full of black dresses and suits.

## Partying **in your 60s and beyond**

• If you have it, you can show your cleavage, but cover your upper arms.
• Wear a colored satin, sheer, or burnout top with a skirt or pants.
• Go for comfort with velvet pumps.
• Invest in an elegant silk skirt or wide-legged pants to which you add a matching top, or alternate with evening knitwear.

Outfits made in soft, colorful silks are flattering and easy and comfortable to wear, while separates are a great investment and can be worn in many different ways— both during the day and in the evening.

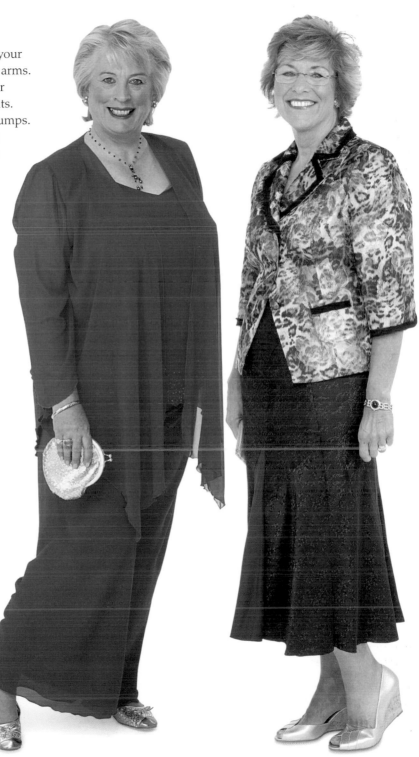

# Index

# Acknowledgments

Staying younger for longer is a subject close to our hearts as we celebrate our joint 118th birthday! No surgery for us—just enthusiasm for what we do, wearing the right clothes and a huge amount of support and patience from our nearest and dearest. Thank you, you know who you are.

Huge thanks go to Katy Denny for championing this book and to Camilla Davis with the Hamlyn team for juggling text and photography so brilliantly.

Thank you to Sue Trevaskis—**colour me beautiful** trainer and award-winning consultant, and our very own expert on hair, whose brain we picked when it came to writing about hairstyle and color.

All our thanks to our stars—and **colour me beautiful** consultants—who beam with confidence in this book: Jo Allen, Paula Cornwell, Caroline Cunningham, Andrea Burgess, Ann Day, Esme Hilliard, Anji Jones, Sylvia Lane, Anne Macfarlane, Franca McBarron, Sylvia Rattenbury, Maria Sadler and her mother Sally Roginski, Shirley Smith, and Christine Southam. They certainly wear the right colors and styles in and out of the photographic studio; they were all unanimously enthusiastic to share their wardrobe on the shoot and are proof that there is life after the big 4–0, 5–0, and certainly the big 6–0.

Of course, this book would not have happened without all the help and support from Audrey Hanna and Fiona Wellins, who not only shadowed us on those hectic preshoot weeks, but who also held the fort in the office when we closeted ourselves away to put this baby to bed. And as usual, Louise Ravenscroft kept a beady eye on our grammar and spelling.

And a big thank you to each other, too. Oh! We laughed and laughed and no doubt increased our laughter lines in the process.

**Pat Henshaw and Veronique Henderson**

## Clothes and accessories acknowledgments

**Artigiano** www.artigiano.co.uk
**Betty Barclay** www.bettybarclay.co.uk
**Chantelle** www.chantelle.com
**Gil Bret** www.gilbret.co.uk
**Sahara** www.saharalondon.com
**Silhouette** www.silhouette.com
**Spirit of the Andes** www.spiritoftheandes.co.uk
**Spirito** www.spirito.co.uk
**Vera Mont** www.veramont.co.uk
**Wall** www.wall-london.com

For more information on services, products and how to become a consultant, contact **colour me beautiful**:

**UK and Headquarters for Europe, Africa and the Middle East**
66 The Business Centre, 15–17 Ingate Place, London SW8 3NS
www.colourmebeautiful.co.uk
info@cmb.co.uk
t: +44 (0)20 7627 5211
f: +44 (0)20 7627 5680

**China** www.qixincolor.com
**Finland** www.colourmebeautiful.fi
**Ireland** www.cmbireland.com
**Hong Kong** www.colourmebeautiful.hk
**Netherlands, Germany, and Belgium**
    www.colourmebeautiful.nl
**Norway** www.colormebeautiful.no
**Slovenia** www.cmb.si
**South Africa** www.colormebeautiful.co.za
**Spain** www.colormebeautifulespaña.com
**Sweden** www.colormebeautiful.se
**USA** www.colourmebeautiful.com

## Picture acknowledgments

All photographs © **Octopus Publishing Group Limited**/Mike Prior apart from the following:

**Alamy** 60, 72, 95. **Camera Press**/Mark Stewart 50; /Theodore Wood 34. **Corbis UK Ltd** 58, 66, 79; /John Feingersh 91; /Jutta Klee 112; /Lisa O'Connor 147; /Tim Pannell 94, 151; /Rune Hellestad 42; /Rainer Holz 148; /Steve Sands 50; /Tim Pannell 94, 151. **Famous** 142. **Getty Images** 86; /Bryan Bedder 34; /Ken Chernus 88; /Kevin Winter 16; /Lenora Gim 132; /Mary Grace Long 106; /MJ Kim 144; /Siri Stafford 67; /Soren Hald 93; /Stephen Shugerman 16. **istockphoto.com** 70. **Masterfile** 92. **Octopus Publishing Group Limited**/Andy Komorowski 99, 105; /Ruth Jenkinson 113. **PA Photos** 145 146, 142. **Photolibrary** 96. **Retna** 58. **Rex Features** 10, 11, 11, 26, 42.

## For Hamlyn

**Executive Editor**  Katy Denny
**Editor**  Camilla Davis
**Executive Art Editor**  Joanna MacGregor and Mark Stevens
**Designer**  Miranda Harvey
**Picture Researcher**  Sarah Smithies and Joanne Forrest Smith
**Senior Production Controller**  Manjit Sihra
**Illustrator**  Jill Bay
**Photographer**  Mike Prior